Sports Supplements for Fitness: How to use them.

Creatine, Glutamine, Whey Protein, energy drinks and more

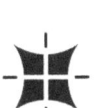

Dager Aguilar Avilés.
United States of America. 2016

Author: Dager Aguilar Aviles
Editing and proofreading: Dager Aguilar Aviles
Cover design: Włodzimierz Wielogórski
Edited by Honoris American-project
Book Layout: Dager Aguilar Aviles

About this edition:
© Dager Aguilar Aviles, 2016
© Ed. Honoris American-project
Sports Supplements for Fitness: How to use them.
ISBN-13:978-1535495325
ISBN-10:1535495324

Precisely for this reason, you must strive to add virtue to your faith; add understanding to your virtue; add self-control in your understanding; add constancy to your self-control; add devotion to God to your constancy; add brotherly affection to your devotion to God; and add to your brotherly affection much love.

2.Pedro 1:5-7

Introduction

The book you have in your hands is a manual for those who regularly conduct training in the gym or other sports. In this book we provide some useful tips on proper use of sports supplements such as creatine, L-carnitine, Whey protein, Omega 3, testosterone, among others. more natural substitutes for each supplement are also proposed. All content exposed here has been corroborated by reliable bibliographical sources and reviewed by experts and specialists in the field. In the pages of this book the reader will find exact recommendations on how to consume each supplement during, before or after training or completing the corresponding cycles of supplementation depending on the finality of his activity in the gym (bodybuilding or fitness).

Here it is not intended to belittle the need for a proper diet, but rather attempts to explain how to supplement the deficits of the daily diet with supplementation of natural origin. For these reasons I speak in this book about the major mistakes that athletes make during sports supplementation.

Theme I: Differences between bodybuilding and fitness to consider before using sports supplements.

The issue of sports supplements is very important for those who consume them. For these reasons, all studies addressing this topic should be initiated by a basic distinction that you, as a reader, should know. We are referring to the difference between fitness and bodybuilding. Keep in mind this difference is very important because the athlete can better define the purpose of his supplementation and also it can determine the level of intensity of supplementation. By this idea we mean that if you want to go to the gym and you will start a complete cycle of training and supplementation, you should be very clear in your mind about what you want to become: fitness or body building. To be clear about this idea, we explain the following 5 most important differences between bodybuilding and fitness.[1]

1-The fitness is for those who mainly want to lose body fat without gaining excessive muscle volume, but may depend on each case. This sport is more focused on getting the perfect combination of size, weight, aesthetics and functionality while bodybuilding focuses more on getting a definition and a volume of muscles with extreme symmetry, sacrificing a maximum percentage of functionality. Usually men should lose body fat to reach at least 8-6% and 10-12% at least in the case of women.

2- Bodybuilding is done by those who want to increase their body mass quite considerably, keeping the body fat levels below 10%, but in some cases can reach 2-4% in high-level professional competitions.

---

[1] These differences were Taken from Padrón, Pablo: seven basic differences between bodybuilding and fitness (in Spanish). Published in Realfitness.es. November 19, 2012. Consulted July, 19, 2016.

3- The fitness training aims at the integral development of all the physical qualities of the athlete: a cardiovascular workout for developing aerobic endurance, training with loads to enhance the muscular system and body exercises that enhance flexibility; all accompanied by a proper and balanced diet and taking proper supplementation in each particular case. The above mentioned allows the person to improve the cardiovascular endurance, flexibility, muscular strength and endurance, agility and balance, brings more speed, toning, and improves physical constitution providing longevity, quality of life and beauty.

4- Because in bodybuilding the people seek an extreme massiveness, understanding it like longer periods of training to get major volume and consuming much higher amounts of calories and protein to maintain and further develop the muscle mass. It is also common consumption of drugs (anabolic androgenic steroids, HGH, insulin, metformin, SERM, DNP, etc.) usually high doses and long cycles, even at the highest professional levels, practically all year. This also happens in the fitness and other sports, but in bodybuilding is quite pronounced. However, there are also natural bodybuilding and fitness competitions where the sports authorities make doping controls, only in pre-contest or throughout the year.

5- The weight of a body fitness is usually between 70 and 85 kilograms defined for a person of average height. Instead, the weight of a bodybuilder is usually between 90 and 105 kilograms defined for a person of average height.

Once clarified some of these differences between fitness and bodybuilding we are able to start with the study of sports supplements and the best ways of consumption.

Theme II: Sports supplements, definition and usefulness

The topic of sports supplements and how to consume them is very controversial. On one side are those who believe that the consumption of sports supplements is correct and, on the other hand, there are people who believe that the consumption of these supplements is negative. The first group have opinion that with the proper advice from experts and medical specialists is possible to achieve excellent results. The second group believe that sports supplements cause long-term damage to the functioning of the body.

Specialists have understood the *sports supplements* as any additional and necessary helps for a sporting activity; this means, any additional aid for the exercise of the body. It is for these reasons that sports supplements are classified into several groups by specialists. On one side is the mechanical supplementation. Mechanical supplementation are all instruments and products used externally to increase body resistance and achieve a pleasurable effect of sporting activity. An example can be sneakers, backpacks, bags and other items used during training.

Other way of supplementation is the pharmaceutical. This group includes anabolic steroids and those supplements produced within the chemical industry. Nutritional supplementation is another important type of supplementation. It refers to system and type of food diets used to increase endurance of the athlete during exercise sections in the gym. The last type of supplementation is known as psychological supplementation. This takes place in the framework of sport psychology. This type of supplementation is based on the idea that all who play sports need excellent psychological conditions. An example can be to have a high concentration during sporting activity. For these reasons the sport and fitness should be seen as a means of reflection, meditation and fun. In this way the gym becomes a method of mental, physical development and increased health.

Sports supplements have several benefits that are important to consider:

1- *They cover the nutritional requirements of the body.* In this case the supplements provide the body with nutrients, proteins and amino acids. This is because during sporting activity the body loses a lot of energy and recovery requires more nutrients than usual. Thus, supplementation should be corresponding to the intensity of the exercise at the gym.

2. *They provide direct physiological support.* An obvious example is the use of creatine.

3- *The third benefit is the pleasurable effect.* This is because the use of sports supplements can contribute to mental stability and mental pleasure during sports activity.

Sports supplements can cause problems at the same time. For these reasons we propose some possible problems:

1- High cost of adquisicion of supplements . In this sense we must be aware that the chemical industry has a very high production cost and always tries to obtain the greatest possible profit from the sale of products. In this sense, distributors and stores also increase prices, but even more for their profits. It is for these reasons that we recommend to all who regularly consume sports supplements make monthly accounting of supplementation spending. We also recommend replacing pharmaceutical supplements for other natural supplements every certain period of time.

2- The second problem of sports supplementation are *the negative effects*. This is an important issue for everyone, but especially for young people. Among young people there is a fairly large group attending the gym for the first time and have not experience on how to handle this activity. Generally these people observe others and try to learn from them, but the risk is when they take sports supplements in large quantities without expert advice because they think that by increasing the dose of consumption will develop faster the body. It is then that the negative effects are manifested. During adolescence, when the body is in full hormonal development, excess supplementation can leave sequels forever. A fairly common example is the excessive consumption of creatine. This excess can cause kidney disorders, problems in the functioning of the liver, abundant diarrhea, severe dehydration, etc. However, we will talk about these issues in the chapter referred to creatine.

3- Another problem in sports supplementation is *inadvertent doping*.[2] This

---

[2] Doping: Consumption of stimulants used to achieve higher efficiency in sports competitions.

happens when stimulants supplements are consumed without knowing that a doping test may be positive due to consumption of these specific supplements. Inadvertent doping can happen because athletes consume supplements without first learn about the possible results in a doping test. Sometimes it happens that athletes look for information about doping on the product before buying it, but the product does not report it and anyway, they decide to buy it. This last situation can happen because of negligence or intent of the supplement producers.

4- Another controversial effect is *the loss of sporting priorities*. To understand this idea we must proceed from the fact that the purpose of sports supplementation is to contribute to athletic efficiency. For these reasons, supplements are used as a supplement to the basic diet and not as main diet. With this idea we mean that It is a huge mistake the complete replacement of basic foods in our diet such as chicken, vegetables, fish and milk for sports supplements. For example, 10 chicken eggs provide the body with approximately 75 g of pure protein. Ingesting of this amount of chicken eggs always be more beneficial and natural than ingestion of 75g of protein chemically processed. Whenever we have the opportunity to choose our diet and supplementation it is recommended to give priority to natural foods and leave supplements as a complementary option. This is the idea and perspective that should never miss in athletes who regularly go to the gym. We must also clarify that the replacement of a section of exercises in the gym by consuming supplements in large quantities is a serious mistake and does not mean that we will automatically develop our body. We say this because it is very common to find people who decide one day not to go to the gym to train and They think that consuming double ration of supplements for that day can achieve the same effect of an exercise section.

Specialists have classified people into four main groups taking into account the different positive and negative effects of ingestion of sports supplements and the purposes for which people ingest these supplements. However, according to the aim of this book, we will focus on the group one of this classification. On the one hand, group 1 is composed of all those who want to change their physical composition or physical image and, on the other hand, there are those who simply want to increase their physical resistance. According to this Group 1 sports supplements are sub-divided into four groups at the same time:

Group A: This is the group that really brings benefits to athletes who consume these supplements. This is because it is known which are the benefits that these supplements provide to the body and these results are scientifically proven. In this group we can find pre-workout energy drinks, energy drinks intended to consume during training and post-workout energy drinks. It is very important that the athlete check if the energy drink that will consume comprises between 5-7% carbohydrate. If the athlete drinks a beverage with more than 7% carbohydrate, the force exerted during training and acid concentration will cause severe stomach aches and constant desire to defecate. Surely this situation hinders the concentration of the athlete and efficiency. If we want to gain weight or muscle mass these energy drinks can be useful because they provide a certain amount of calories and allow stability of blood glucose levels. It is in this way that you can avoid the mental and physical fatigue. On the other hand, if you want to lose weight we recommend less consumption of energy drinks; thus the excess calories in the body is prevented. In this case the energy drink consumed should not exceed 5% carbohydrate. Another supplement that is part of this group is the protein. Protein is needed to build muscle, but there is a point where it loses all its usefulness and becomes something dangerous. That is why protein supplements should be consumed at the right time and in the right quantities. Experts believe that the whey protein is one of the best supplements because is easily absorbed by the human body, but they always recommend combining whey protein with simple carbohydrates to intensify the absorption by the body. On the other hand we can find the protein casein. Casein protein differs from the whey protein because it has a slower absorption in the human body. It is why a lot of athletes prefer to consume whey protein before bed. Other supplements of this group are gels for athletes. These are useful because it increases the strength, elasticity and hydration. However, excess consumption of gels can cause gastrointestinal disorders and intolerance. In this group A are also important candy bars for athletes. These are useful because are provides with vitamins, minerals and often they have creatine. But we recommend that the athlete should always observe the amount of vitamins and minerals contained in each product before buy it because many times the amount of vitamins and minerals is so little that is insignificant. Thus, there are many supplements in this group such as glutamine, omega 3, amino acids and more, but these mentioned before are the most popular among athletes and of easier acquisition.

Group B: In group B are sports supplements with known benefits, but still they have not been scientifically proven. Therefore it requires more scientific research.

Group C: In this group are sports supplements that do not bring any benefits to the human body; but even so, are often sold in many stores of sports supplements for athletes. To get an idea we can say that 80% of supplements currently sold in stores are classified in this group and in group D.

Group D: In this group are all those legally prohibited supplements and those considered as doping supplements.

In this book we will focus mainly on supplements of Group A

Theme III: Creatine

Creatine was discovered in 1832 by French chemist Michel Eugène Chevreul. In 1847, Lieberg concluded that the accumulation of creatine in the body is directly related to the production of muscular work. This research was conducted by comparing the amount of creatine in muscles of wild foxes respect to domestic foxes. Thus it was found that wild foxes possessed ten times more creatine in muscles than domestic foxes. Many experts believe the first to use creatine as a sports supplement were athletes from the former Soviet Union in the 1960s. Since the use of creatine has become popular. To get an idea we can say that the Olympic Games in Atlanta (1996) were popularly known as "creatine games". Nevertheless, creatine is not among the substances prohibited by the International Olympic Committee, but many experts believe that the use of creatine in Olympic competitions and high level is anti-thetical.

Creatine is produced naturally in the human body, especially in the kidneys and liver. It is produced from amino acids and is transported through the blood. Approximately 95% of the creatine in the body is concentrated in skeletal muscle.[3] Creatine is not an essential nutrient because is synthesized from L-arginine and L-methionine.[4] It is important to note that in humans and animals half of the stored creatine is obtained from the consumption of meat. This happens because vegetables do not have creatine and that is why vegetarians have low levels of muscle creatine. Nevertheless, they can increase their muscle creatine levels if they consume creatine supplements.[5] The enzyme GATM (L-arginine: glycine amidinotransferase

---

[3] «Creatine». MedLine Plus Supplements. U.S. National Library of Medicine. 20 de julio de 2010. Consultado el 3 de enero de 2015 a las 01:34hrs.

[4] GREENHALF, P. L.. INT J.:Creatine and Its application as an ergogenic aid"; Sports Nutr., 15(Sup to 5), 100-110. 1995.

[5] BURKE DG, CHILIBECK PD, PARISE G, CANDOW DG, MAHONEY D, TARNOPOLSKY M (2003): «Effect of creatine and weight training on muscle creatine and performance in vegetarians». Medicine and science in sports and exercise 35 (11): 1946–55.

(EC 2.1.4.1) is a mitochondrial enzyme and is responsible for catalyzing the first rate-limiting step in the biosynthesis of creatine. This process takes place mainly in the kidney and pancreas.[6] The second enzyme involved in the biosynthesis process of creatine is GAMT (Guanidinoacetate N-methyltransferase, EC: 2.1.1.2 EC: 2.1.1.2), primarily expressed in the liver and pancreas.[7] There are genetic deficiencies in the biosynthetic pathway of creatine that lead to different severe neurological defects.[8] So it is advisable to check with medical specialists if our body is conditioned to consume creatine as a sports supplement. It is known that a person having a weight of 70kg can retain approximately 120 g of creatine.[9] The purpose of storage of creatine in the body is the creation of phosphocreatine (PCr). Phosphocreatine is formed by mixing creatine with phosphorus and, in the process, ATP is

---

[6] «ETH ETH E-Collection: *Methylglyoxal, creatine and mitochondrial micro-compartments - ETH E-Collection*». E-collection.ethbib.ethz.ch. 19 de abril de 2008.
[7] *Ibidem.*
[8] «L-Arginine:Glycine Amidinotransferase». Ncbi.nlm.nih.gov
[9] BEMBEN, M. & LAMONT, H. D.:*"Creatine Supplementation and exercise performance"*. Sport Med., 35(2), 107-125. 2005.

consumed. ATP(adenosine triphosphate) is present in muscle cells and creatine kinase too,[10] but as the muscles are not able to synthesize the creatine do not have another option that take the needed creatine from the bloodstream. The important thing here is to note that the ATP is the energy constituent of muscle cells. On the other hand, we must note that one of the functions of creatine is to regulate the pH of the cells.

Studies on anaerobic athletes have shown that exercise depletes the creatine in muscle in the first 5-10 seconds of training.[11] This limit is very controversial because other experiments have shown cases where the phosphocreatine and creatine reserves are depleted in the first 20-30 segundos beginning training.[12] The truth is that there is no research that has demonstrated superior limits to one minute since the start of

[10] BARBANY, J.R.:(2002)."*Alimentación para el deporte y la salud"*, Barcelona: Martínez Roca.
[11] MESA, J.L.; GUTIÉRREZ-SAINZ, A. Y CASTILLO, M.J.: (2001)."*Suplementación oral de creatina y rendimiento deportivo*", Lecturas: Educación Física y Deportes, 36.
[12] NACLERIO, F.: (2001). *"Conceptos fundamentales acerca de la creatina como suplemento o integrador dietético"*. Naclerio, F. (2001). Lecturas: Educación Física y Deportes, 30.

training. Consumption of ATP stores in the muscles causes lower levels of phosphocreatine and, consequently, muscle fatigue occurs. This phenomenon is expressed in muscle stiffness, severe muscle pain and exhaustion of muscle strength. So we recommend to the athlete when he has these symptoms rest the muscle until recovery became the best option. Many athletes think that when it comes to muscle fatigue the best option is to consume more sports supplements and this is a serious mistake; that is why we reiterate that the best option is to let the muscle resting until recovery. Anyway, there are sports supplements in these cases that help to catalyze the recovery of the affected muscle, but consumption of these supplements is effective only during the muscle resting period. In this way, Creatine intake causes phosphocreatine reserves are not depleted quickly and you can work out at the gym for a longer period.[13]

---

[13] KREIDER, R.B.; FERREIRA, M. Y WILSON, M. (1998).: *"Effects of creatine supplementation on body composition, strength and sprint perfomance"* en *Medicine and Science in Sports and Exercise*, 31, 1770-1777.

ATP levels remain relatively high when we perform high intensity anaerobic efforts for more than 5s and even 30s. This means that ATP levels do not descend more than 40% -60% compared to their initial values. But nevertheless, phosphocreatine decreases considerably until very low levels.[14] As well as we said before, creatine is transported through the bloodstream, but that transportation is possible thanks to a carrier protein who needs chlorine and sodium to achieve that process. we are talking about the crea-T (very similar to dopamine). Studies on creatine consumption by aerobic athletes have shown that there are few ergogenic effects[15] on the development and performance of these sports. This is because the demand and consumption of metabolic energy is no longer dependent on creatine, but it depends on other sources: lipids or glycogen consumption. This process is known as *aerobic glycolysis*.

---

[14] WARRNER, J. P., THARRION, W. J., PATTON, J. F., CAHMPAGNE, C. M., MITOTTI, P. & LIEBERMAN, H.. J. : "*The effects of creatine monhudrate supplementation on obstacle course and multiple bench press performance*", Strength Cond. Res. 16(500-508.). 2002
[15] That causes or increases muscle power.

Previously we had said that creatine is present in meat, but the best meat to eat in this regard is the fish. We particularly recommend the herring and salmon, although milk products and eggs are also rich in creatine.[16] Creatine is also found in some vegetables, but in very small quantities. We recommend always to consume creatine supplementation accompanied by a auxiliary diet of carbohydrates and amino acids because then the transportation of the ATP to cells is potentiated, the glycemic index grows, insulin secretion is stimulated and, finally, creatine is taken up by the cellular tissues in a better way. Several research on creatine uptake by insulin[17] show that the greater effectiveness of this process occurs in the first 24 hours after training. [18] After

---

[16] *"American College of Sport Medicine"*. Round Table, the physiological and health effects of oral creatine supplementation. Med. Sci. Sports Exc., 32(3), 706-717. 2000.

[17] SNOW, R. J. & MURPHY, R. M.: *"Factor Influencing Creatine Loading into human Skeletal Muscle"*,. Exc sports Sci. Rev, 31(3), 154-158. 2003.

[18] WALZEL, B., SPEER, O., BOEHM, E., KRISTIANSEN, S., CHAN, S., CLARKE, K., MAGYAR, J. P., RICHTER, E. A. & WALLIMANN, T.. AM J.: *"New creatine transporter assay and identification of distintict creatine transporter isoforms in muscle"* in Endocrinol Metab, 283, 390-401. 2002.

those 24 hours creatine effectiveness will begin to declining in all the body.

Researchers have also shown that vitamin E helps in the transportation of creatine to muscles.[19] Especially vitamin E is recommended to avoid saturation of creatine in the blood. This shows us that if we consider a good dosage strategy in the consumption of sports supplements we can ensure that the creatine stores in muscles increase by 10-30%.[20]

How to consume creatine?

Creatine can be consumed at any time of the day (seen as sports supplement). Only caffeine can affect the absorption of creatine in the body, so it is not recommended to drink it with coffee or drinks that contain caffeine. Nevertheless, researches on this issue of caffeine have not been

---

[19] RICO-SANZ, J.: (1997). *"Efectos de suplementación de creatina en el metabolismo muscular y energético",* en Archivos de Medicina del Deporte, 61, 391-396.
[20] SNOW, R. J. & MURPHY, R. M.: Ob cit.

entirely convincing.[21] However experts have shown in several experiments that not everybody has the same capacity of absorption of creatine; even, there are athletes who are completely intolerant to creatine.[22] It has also been shown that people with higher absorption of creatine are those who had lower levels of creatine before begin treatment of supplementation. A very clear example are vegetarians.[23]

It is very important that the consumer of creatine knows that effects depend on the levels of growth of intramuscular creatine. This means that if the total intramuscular creatine levels are high then all doses consumed by the athlete should be according with that fact and, only in this way, the expansion of creatine in muscles will be faster and

[21] K. VANDENBERGHE, N. GILLIS, M. VAN LEEMPUTTE, P. VAN HECKE, F. VANSTAPEL AND P. HESPEL: *"Caffeine counteracts the ergogenic action of muscle creatine loading"*, in Journal of Applied Physiology, Vol 80, Issue 2 452-457, 1996

[22] SYROTUIK, D. & BELL, G. J. J. STRENGTH : *"Acute creatine monohydrate supplementation: A descriptive physiological profile of responders vs nonresonders"*, Cond. Res.. 18(3), 610-617. 2004.

[23] GREENHALF, P. L.. INT J.: *Creatine and Its application as an ergogenic aid"*; Sports Nutr., 15(Sup to 5), 100-110. 1995.

more effective. But if our muscles have a high absorption capacity of creatine not will need high doses of supplementation. When we consume more creatine than necessary the body will expel the excess through urine and only will consume the amount he needs. As a result of this irresponsibility only we will get severe damage to our renal system.

The traditional way of administration of creatine for normal people is divided into two phases: the first one is known as "initial phase" and can last between five or six days. The second phase is known as "maintenance phase" and is extended by about two months. The third phase is known as "resting phase". This phase also is extended during two months. Currently there is much controversy about the amount of grams that a person should consume at each phase. Most experts recommend that during the first phase a person should consume 1 g of creatine per 10 kilogram of body weight each day. However in the second phase it is recommended to consume a quarter of amount that was consumed during the first phase.[24] Really it depends on the purpose of the person attending the gym because if this person wants to increase the size of his muscles quickly should perform Phase 1 and 2 below, but if the purpose is to improve metabolic efficiency will be better to make a single dose for at least a month. Why only one time at month.? Well, when creatine is administered at a rate of 20g daily for several days 30% of the administered creatine is absorbed by the body in the first two days, but after the second day will be absorbed only 15% of the creatine supplied to our body.[25] After the cessation of intake of creatine a person will need about 30 days to return to previous levels at the start of supplementation.[26]

The pure creatine causes great instability in the body, so it is easy to find as monohydrate in

[24] RAWSON, E. S. & VOLEK, J. S. J.: *"Effects of creatine Supplementation and Resistance Training on Muscle Strength and Weightlifting Performance"*, Strength Cond. Res. 17(4), 822-831. 2003.

[25] CHANUTIN A.: "The fate of creatine when administered to man". *J Biol Chem 1926; 67: 29-37.*

[26] HULTMAN E, SÖDERLUND K, TIMMONS JA, ET AL., *J APPL PHYSIOL*: *"Muscle creatine loading in men".* 1996; 81: 232-7

powder form. The creatine also can be provided intravenously, but this variant is only utilized in hospitals for cardiovascular surgeries. In many stores is also possible to find other variants of creatine like creatine citrate and phosphocreatine. The difference between these presentations of creatine is focused on the concentration of the compound because the creatine citrate molecule contains 40% of creatine and phosphocreatine 62.3%. The pure creatine before being consumed must be dissolved in liquids such as water, tea or fruit juice. When creatine is diluted in water or other liquid is beneficial to add a little sugar because insulin in the sugar facilitates the absorption of creatine.[27] We remind you not to mix creatine with drinks that have caffeine because caffeine tends to slow down the process of absorption of creatine in the body.

Because creatine has low stability in water we must always consume it immediately after dissolving. The best times to consume creatine

---

[27] SNOW, R. J. & MURPHY, R. M.: Ob.cit.

are during the main meals because it is in those moments when insulin levels rise. During the period of creatine supplementation it is very important to drink a lot of water, especially if we consider that the oral delivery of creatine between 1 and 10g requires at least 2hrs to reach the maximum level of concentration in blood. Also, when higher doses are consumed, this process can take up to three hours.[28] Water greatly facilitates the process of absorption of creatine and if this supplementation is combined with another supplementation of vitamin E, glutamine and amino acids is even better.

In the case of people who go regularly to the gym and have a very intense training, we recommend them to extend the possibility to extend the phase 1 and 2 of creatine supplementation up to four months. The third phase we recommend that lasts at least one month. During this month of rest (third phase), the athlete should make supplementation cycles with glutamine to regenerate muscle; but training in the gym should not be stopped. This

---

[28] PERSKY, A. & BRAZEAU, G. A: Ob.Cit.

issue of keeping training in the gym is very important because exercise and drink lots of water are the main complements of creatine supplementation. Many bodybuilders prefer to consume a dose of creatine 30 minutes before going to the gym and we think that is very beneficial for those who do intense workouts, so it is quite usual that many trainers recommend this technique to athletes.

Experts say there are no known cases of illness in people who have used creatine for two months uninterruptedly, but at the same time, there are no reports on studies respect to this rhythm of supplementation of creatine in longer periods.[29] Finally we recommend that if the athlete does not have whey protein to drink after training in the gym can consume a small dose of creatine to stimulate muscle recovery.

---

[29] MELVIN H. WILLIAMS: *"Creatine Supplementation and Exercise Performance: An Update";* Journal of the American College of Nutrition, Vol. 17, No. 3, 216-234 (1998).

Effects of creatine consumption

The effects of creatine consumption can be divided into two: positive and negative. Among positive effects we can find:[30]

1- *Higher performance in intense exercises and short term exercises.*

Creatine molecule acts as a reserve for the regeneration of ATP. When the athlete begins intense physical exercises and short term exercises, muscle receives energy from ATP. If we consume the correct doses of creatine before starting training in the gym, will be guaranteed an increase of ATP production by 30%. At the same time has been shown how increases production of phosphocreatine by 20%. Also it showed that after 15 days of supplementation with creatine when the

---

[30] Loreferido a los efectos positivos de la creatina ha sido tomado del sitio web infocreatina.com. obtenible en http://www.infocreatina.com/efectos. Consultado el 3 de enero de 2016 a las 04:33hrs.

process of suplemmentation was suspended, concentration in muscle was higher compared to the initial amounts.

2- Decreasing muscle fatigue

Creatine consumption reduces muscle fatigue when series repetitions are performed with great intensity and in a short time because in this way reduces ammonium levels in body and descends intracellular pH and blood pH too. This process is ultimately expressed in reduction in the acidity and increased muscle strength.

3- Significant increase in strength

Of the preceding paragraphs it is easily understood that when we consume creatine we get more energy and that is translated into greater endurance, strength and efficiency in training.

4- Promotes increased muscle mass

Creatine causes an increase of the volume of the cells due to water retention within them. This situation causes simultaneously cell regeneration and hypertrophy and facilitates protein synthesis during the recovery periods of physical activity.

5-*Increases the speed of transfer of substrates*

Creatine increases the transfer rate between substrates of the cellular compartments such as mitochondria and cytoplasm. These processes streamline ATP recovery during the pause periods.

6- *Accelerates muscle contraction and relaxation*

the creatine consumption accelerates muscle contraction and relaxation because facilitates the release of calcium from the sarcoplasmic reticulum Cell. In this process actomyosin bridges are separated faster and muscle fiber is stimulated again and increases the frequency and efficiency of training in the gym.

With respect to the negative effects of creatine consumption we must bear in mind that there is no evidence that creatine really affects the renal system.[31] However there is controversy among researchers regarding the influence of consumption of creatine in body weight gain (due to the anabolic function of creatine) and increased muscle glycogen. These effects have been demonstrated in men, but there are no proven studies on women.[32] The effects of weight gain is attributed to fluid retention, but there is no hard evidence about it. Also many doctors have reported cases in which the intake of creatine has

---

[31] KURT A PLINE: *"The Effect of Creatine Intake on Renal Function"*, The Annals of Pharmacotherapy: Vol. 39, No. 6, pp. 1093-1096.

[32] GONZÁLEZ BOTO, R.; GARCÍA LÓPEZ, D. Y HERRERO ALONSO, J.A.: (2003)."*La suplementación con creatina en el deporte y su relación con el rendimiento deportivo*",. Revista Internacional de Medicina y Ciencias de la Actividad Física y el Deporte, vol. 3 (12) pp. 242-259.

caused stomach disorders. Example, very watery diarrhea and muscle cramps, but there are no sensitive evidence demonstrating their causes.[33] The New England Journal of Medicine[34] has been reported that creatine consumption, sometimes, changes the character and emotional temperament and, for these reasons, before starting supplementation, the athlete must seek advice by professionals on proper dosage that should be better for him. They also recommend medical checkup and performing additional tests at regular intervals during the period of supplementation and then also. It is highly recommended to consume at least 1.5 liters of liquid daily during the period of creatine supplementation because there have been many cases of people swoon, dehydrated or with constipation due to excessive fluid retention caused by the additional creatine. That is why we also recommend that when the athlete does creatine supplementation should go to the gym

---

[33] *"American College of Sport Medicine"*. Round Table, the physiological and health effects of oral creatine supplementation. Med. Sci. Sports Exc., 32(3), 706-717. 2000.
[34] v.rol. 340:814-815 n.10

and train hard to process any additional creatine. You should always remember that it is a serious mistake add creatine as supplement to our body without performing regular exercise. This is fairly common in teenagers who want to gain weight thinking that because of intake creatine, without regular exercise, will increase their weight quickly. Finally, we note that in March 2015 the British Journal of Cancer found a possible link between the consumption of supplements containing creatine and testicular cancer.[35] Hence the importance of not exceed the correct dose during creatine supplementation.

35

http://www.nature.com/bjc/journal/v112/n7/full/bjc201526a.html

Theme IV: Glutamine

Glutamine is created in the human body when glutamic acid decomposes and is mixed with ammonia molecules that contain nitrogen. We can think of it as a kind of sponge of nitrogen. Then, when glutamine absorbs ammonia the nitrogen is sent between tissues. In this way the nitrogen is used by the body for tissue repair and cell growth. Several studies have shown that between 30 and 35% of all nitrogen used in the human body comes from the breakdown of protein which is transported in the form of glutamine. Glutamine molecule can also be divided to re-synthesize glutamic acid or glutamate and thus becomes a critical source of ammonia and nitrogen. Experts believe that approximately 70% of glutamine in our body is produced in skeletal muscle and from there moves to the small intestine, kidneys and White blood cells. It is at these points where the increased use of glutamine is concentrated. Internal levels of this amino acid depend on several factors. For example, pregnancy and lactation significantly deplete the body deposits, as strenuous exercise, illness, fasting, rapid growth and development and other physiological conditions of extreme stress. Therefore in these conditions intake glutamine supplementation is very appropriate.[36]

Food of animal origin are an essential source of this amino acid. Eggs, pork and chicken are among the foods with highest concentration of glutamine, but also raw meat and turkey are rich in glutamine. The most recommended fish is salmon. It is recommended that these foods are consumed in the most natural way as possible, thinking on possibility that many of these animals were fed with hormones and other chemicals. Dairy products are also an important source of glutamine and among them are relevant milk, yogurt and fresh cheeses. Others glutamine-rich

---

[36] Taked from *glutamine.org*. Consultado el 3 de enero de 2016 a las 04:55hrs.

foods are vegetables, especially spinach, cabbage and parsley. We also recommend eat all these vegetables in raw to make better use of their properties. Also legumes and whole grains are recommended for their high concentration of glutamine.[37]

Glutamine is one of the few amino acid molecules having two nitrogen atoms (Normally only have one N atom). These characteristics give a privileged position to glutamine in the body's metabolic activities because the proportion of nitrogen facilitates the body metabolic processes. Biosynthesis of glutamine in the body cleans high concentrations of ammonia in the brain and consequently the ammonia is moved to other parts of the body, but at lower concentrations. Glutamine is also used by the body in the biosynthesis of glutathione oxidant and in protein synthesis because it is found in large amounts in the muscles and blood.[38] Other relevant

---

[37] PHYLLIS A. BALCH, AVERY: *"Prescription for Nutritional Healing"* , 2006

[38] Glutamine in the muscles occupies almost 60% of the amino acids

importance of glutamine is that it levels in the blood are indicators of possible catabolic disorders, for instance, intestinal necrosis.

Glutamine has a tampon effect which neutralizes the excess of acid in the muscles. This excess is usually generated by the practice of intense exercise. The most obvious example is lactic acid. This is very important because many people do not know that this excess acid concentration is the root cause of muscle fatigue and muscular catabolic. This tampon effect is manifested in decreasing of the positively charge of H + ions that arrived from acids.[39] Some studies have shown that consumption of glutamine causes an additional tampon capacity when the muscular balance (acid/alkaline) breaks to create more acid.[40] Thus, thanks to the buffering effect, greater intensity and efficiency is achieved in training. It has also been scientifically proven that glutamine

---

[39] *"Increased plasma bicarbonate and growth hormone after an oral glutamine load",* Welbourne, T.C. Am J Clin Nutr, 61: 1058-61, 1995.
[40] WELBOURNE, T.C., & JOSHI, S.: *"Interorgan glutamine metabolism during acidosis",* Jnl Parent Ent Nutr, 14: 775-855, 1990.

prevents loss of muscle mass during standing time or during the time of intense exercise. Glutamine plays an important role in renal tubule cells because with glutaminase synthesizes the ammonia.

How to consume glutamine?

Glutamine is a semi-essential amino acid to prevent stress, trauma and infections and it can be used in those cases where a person has been bedridden for long periods. Also cancer patients and AIDS consume glutamine, but athletes frequently use it for muscle recovery.[41] This happen because when we live under stress, trauma or surgery, our muscles segregate glutamine into the bloodstream and because of this they lose weight significantly. supplementation of L-Glutamine may be beneficial in cases of arthritis, immune deficiency diseases, fibrosis, intestinal disorders, peptic ulcers, radiation damage, cancer, etc.

---

[41] "Prescription for Nutritional Healing", Phyllis A. Balch, Avery, 2006

Glutamine is sold in powder form and capsules. It is advisable to keep glutamine supplements in dry places because humidity causes hydrolysis of glutamine into ammonia and pyro-glutamic acid. It is also advisable not to provide to people with any problems related to excess of ammonia in the blood.[42] Several researches in animals have shown that glutamine supplementation can affect appetite but this study has not been proven in humans.[43]

L Glutamine is synthesized by the liver and lungs and certain amounts of glutamine are released during intense exercise. Scientific studies have shown that intensive cycles of exercises consume almost all the natural reserves of glutamine in the muscles and, for this reason, glutamine supplementation is recommended for

---

[42] COOPER, ARTHUR J.L.: *"Role of glutamine in cerebral nitrogen metabolism and ammonia neurotoxicity"*, Mental Retardation and Developmental Disabilities Research Reviews, Volume 7, Issue 4, Pages 280 - 286, 2001

[43] OPARA, E.C., PETRO A., et al.: *"L-glutamine supplementation of a high fat diet reduces body weight and attenuates hyperglycemia and hyperinsulinemia in C57BL/6J mice"*, en J Nutr, 126: 273-79, 1996.

bodybuilders.[44] To have a clear idea we can say that, for example, athletes who perform anaerobic exercise release about 45% of muscle glutamine levels compared to pre-exercise; but, when these athletes continue with aerobic exercise for 10 days, the concentration of glutamine in the plasma drops to 50%. The decrease in glutamine levels are maintained even six days after recovery from exercise. These data suggest that these athletes need glutamine supplementation in their diets able to replenish their muscles. The muscles that are exploited in training (without a suitable replacement of glutamine) increase your risk of infection and often recover more slowly from damages.[45]

Currently, There is much discussion about the dosage and when to take glutamine supplements. Experts feel that supplementation should begin a gradual manner. During this period you should consume small doses and observe the effects on

---

[44] KEAST, D., ARSTEIN, D., ET AL. MED J AUST,: *"Depression of plasma glutamine concentration after exercise stress and its possible influence on the immune system,"*, 162; 15-8, 1995.
[45] *Ibídem.*

the body and the reactions of your body. As always we recommend be assisted by a specialist to periodically evaluate the effects on your body. The most experts consider that If you are training regularly at gym should drink between 5-15 grams per day (1 gram per 10kg of muscle) divided into two or three doses over twenty-four hours. The most popular times to take them are in the morning, before and after training, and just before going to sleep. Research conducted so far do not suggest the need to establish cycles for supplementation with glutamine or differentiate between a charging period and maintenance.[46] How to take glutamine depends on the format in which you consume. If you have tablets or pills, you can drink it with a little water or fruit juice. If it is in the form of powders, you can do the same or add it to your protein shake. It may be a good idea to combine glutamine with other substances or nutrients before drinking. First, you can consider the posibility of join glutamine with sodium and other electrolytes because glutamine transport

---

[46] Taken from www.glutamine.org. Consulted on January 3, 2016 at 04: 55hrs.

occurs through a mechanism dependent of sodium and experts have shown that in this way increases much more cell volume, electrolyte absorption and hydration. This will be useful for endurance athletes and bodybuilders because the volume of water in the cell is one of the many determinants of muscle hypertrophy. In addition to sodium, glutamine may be accompanied with elements such as BCAA, which will help to increase muscle mass gains and improve your performance in training.[47] It is advisable to take glutamine when the stomach is empty because, thus, will not interact with other amino acids obtained from the diet.

Effects of Glutamine consumption.

There are many situations where you can get benefits if properly glutamine is consumed and under specialist supervision. These situations are:

a. Under stress
b. Preferential fuel for intestinal cells.

---

[47] Ibidem.

c. Prevents diarrhea and poor absorption of nutrients.

d. When there is muscle trauma or shock.

e. The practice of sport that requires considerable physical effort.

f. When there is a process of recovery from any type of lesion.

g. Intensity workouts.

h. When an infection is detected in muscle or skin.

i. If you have burns.

j. If you have physical exhaustion.

k. Eating disorders that cause muscle catabolism.

l. Certain pathologies or diseases related to the practice of sports.

m. Workouts that require a long endurance.

In general on the positive side effects of glutamine consumption can be found:[48]

---

[48]Everything here refers to all the positive benefits of glutamine was taken from the site glutamine.org. Consulted on January 3, 2016 at 04: 55hrs

1. Construction of muscle

For people who are trying to gain muscle mass, this will be their main advantage. Our muscles are composed largely of glutamine and if we supplement this amino acid, can help us in protein synthesis. When the body has low levels, the working sessions of high intensity can exhaust our muscles and this will cause you get tired faster. So, If you take supplements, you allow your muscles work a little harder and improve your strength. In addition, supplementation supports you in the recovery of muscles after the session. Remember, however, that glutamine alone will not do your muscle grow instantly; to achieve this goal, you need a healthy diet and regular exercise. Glutamine is a supplement, not a miracle pill.

2. Cell volume and hydration.

As glutamine helps our cells to maintain volume and adequate level of hydration can decrease recovery time of wounds and burns, and help repair muscle more effectively

3. Increased growth hormone.

Several studies have shown that glutamine supplementation can drastically increase the levels of growth hormone in the human body. In fact, some research has come to show up to 400% more than normal. This factor can help in different situations. On one hand, the increased production of this hormone increases the metabolic rate. This increase in metabolism causes the people consumers of glutamine becomes able to process more food faster and burn more fat more efficiently. On the other hand, growth hormone is very important to support muscle growth.

4. Power source for your immune system.

It can act as a primary energy source for your immune system. If you have more glutamine, will improve your ability to fight any infection or disease.

5. Gastrointestinal Health

It is absolutely critical in terms of your gastrointestinal health. Over the past two decades, there have been many studies that show how glutamine helps cure problems such as ulcers or leaky gut syndrome, sometimes very quickly. Generally also helps to our digestive system because glutamine is one of the most important nutrients for our intestines.

6. Increased brain function

Being an innate neurotransmitter, glutamine helps pass information between different parts of the brain and improves connection, concentration and attention of the person.

Dietary or nutritional supplements are not regulated and therefore there are no recommendation or prescription by any official agency indicating the ideal dose of glutamine for every purpose and occasion. Thanks to all research and clinical trials, it has been shown that the use of glutamine supplementation does not entail any adverse side effects to our health. However, an excess in the use of this supplement may have no beneficial effects, such as allergic reactions or interactions with prescription drugs. Clearly, you should consult your doctor before beginning any supplementation with glutamine if you have any questions or suffering from any kind of disease. In addition, you should go to him if you experience any of the following serious side effects: blood in the urine or stool, cold hands and feet, circulatory problems, darkening of skin color, heart rate or breathing faster than normal and loss of conscience. Some people may experience an allergic reaction to these types of supplements. The following symptoms are indicative of that kind of reaction: hives, difficulty breathing, chest tightness, swelling of the face, hands, ankles, tongue, mouth and/or throat. The excessive intake of glutamine can also cause the following gastrointestinal side effects: nausea, vomiting, gas, abdominal pain or cramps, diarrhea or constipation. Prolonged diarrhea may be a potential risk of dehydration if the individual does not consume enough liquids to replace lost fluids.[49]

[49] Ibidem.

Theme V: Proteins. Whey Protein.

Proteins are biologically important nutrients. These are macromolecules that constitute the main nutrient for the formation of the body's muscles. Among the key functions of proteins we can find:[50]

- Proteins have a defensive role because they create antibodies against disease-producing pathogens agents. From bacterial toxins, such as snake venom or botulism, are generated proteins with defensive functions. Mucins, for example, protect mucous membranes and has germicidal effect. The Fibrinogen and thrombin contribute in the formation of blood clots to prevent bleeding.

---

[50] Taken from http://proteinas.org.es/funciones-de-las-proteinas website. Retrieved January 3, 2016 at 13: 10hrs.

Immunoglobulins act as antibodies against possible antigens.

- Proteins have other regulatory functions because they are formed by the following compounds: Hemoglobin, plasma proteins, hormones, digestive juices, enzymes and vitamins that cause chemical reactions that occur in the body. Some proteins such as cyclin are useful for regulating the process of cell division and other proteins are useful for regulating the expression of some genes.

- Proteins with enzymatic function are the most specialized and numerous. These act as catalysts to accelerate chemical reactions of metabolism.

- Proteins also function as shock absorbers, keeping stable internal pH and osmotic balance. This capacity is known as homeostatic function of proteins.

- The contraction of muscles through actin and myosin is a function of contractile proteins that facilitate the movement of cells. In this way are constituted the myofibrils which are responsible for muscle contraction. The dynein is also implicated in the contractile protein function because it relates to the movement of cilia and flagella.

- The resistance function or structural function of proteins is also of great importance since proteins form filling and supporting tissues conferring elasticity and resistance to organs and some tissues. Some proteins form cell structures as histones, which are part of the chromosomes that regulate gene expression. Some glycoproteins act as receptors part of cell membranes or facilitate the transport of substances. Proteins also play an energy role for the body because they can provide up to 4 kcal. energy per gram. Examples of the backup function of proteins are the lactalbumin from milk, egg ovalbumin, barley hordein and gliadin from wheat grain. In this way it constitutes the amino acid for embryo development.

- Proteins perform transport functions. Examples include hemoglobin and myoglobin. These proteins carry oxygen in the blood of vertebrate organisms and muscles respectively. Other examples of proteins whose function is to transport electrons are cytochromes and carrying lipoproteins that transport lipids in the blood.

Between protein-rich foods we can find:[51]

- The pork loin: is one of the foods with higher protein content. The pork loin contains 50 grams of protein and only 8 grams of fat per 100 grams. Besides being one of the foods with more protein, the pork

_____
[51] Ibidem.

loin is free of fat so it is highly recommended if you want to follow a low-fat diet and generally and high in protein.

- Soy is a very nutritious vegetable particularly rich in protein. Soy contains a high percentage of high-quality protein, almost 37 grams of protein per 100 grams of soy and also it contains most of the essential amino acids except for methionine, which can be completed by combining with other soy-rich foods such as cereals. If soy is compared in the same waight with other foods we can see that contains twice more protein than meat, 4 times the proteins of one egg and 12 times the protein in milk.

- Skim milk powder also has a high level of protein because it is milk from which has been virtually eliminated all fat, but retains all its proteins. The percentage of normal proteins from skimmed milk powder is 35 grams per 100 grams and contain only one gram of fat per 100; besides a great source of protein, skimmed milk is a good source of vitamin B.

- Cured Manchego cheese is a food rich in protein with 32 grams of protein per 100 but yet has a high content of fat (35 grams). Manchego cheese curds reduces almost in 29% the amount of protein and the fresh Manchego cheese in 26%. This shows that if the cheese is cured less will have less protein. Alternatively, the fat cheese has up to 39% protein and low fat content. Other cheeses such as Edam cheese, Gruyere or Emmental also have a 29% protein. Roquefort cheese has a 23% protein and Cabrales has 21% protein.

- The Cod is a good example of a food rich in protein and low in fat, besides being an important source of vitamins and minerals that make this fish become one of the foods that contain more protein recommended for anyone.

- Serrano ham, with 30.5 grams of protein per 100 grams, is an important source of protein for our body and a good ally in any sports diet. In addition, we must consider the high biological value of proteins of the ham because they are easily assimilated by the body. So, the ham is a food highly valued because is rich in high quality protein.

- The peanut has many properties and also has a considerable amount of protein because per 100g of peanuts we obtain 27 grams of protein. The groundnuts, although have many nutrients and properties, should be eaten in moderation because are heavy to digest.

- Sausages like salami have 25.8 grams of protein per 100 g of weight. In this sense, tuna, turkey breast and Lentils are around 24 grams of protein per 100g weight.

- Other foods with a high percentage of protein are:

1. Lentils (23.5%)
2. Tuna (23% protein for each 100 grams of tuna)
3. peas (23%)
4. Roquefort cheese (23%)
5. chicken breast (22.8%)
6. Fiambre turkey (22.4%)
7. Chorizo, ham (22%)
8. Canned Sardines (22%)
9. non-greasy Pork (21.2%)
10. non-fat beef (21%)
11. Bonito (21h%)
12. Cabrales cheese (21%)
13. Fillet of beef (20.7%)
14. clean beef (20.7%)
15. Grilled chicken (20.6%)
16. Liver (20%)
17. Norway lobster, prawns, shrimp ... (20.1%)
18. • Chickpeas (20%)
19. • Almonds (20%)
20. • Lean pork (20%)

21. • Blood sausage (19.5%)
22. • goatling (19%)
23. • Chick peas, white beans (19%)
24. • salmon (19%)
25. • Lamb (18%)
26. • Pistachios (17.6%)
27. • Bacalao (17%)
28. • semi-fatty pork (16.7%)
29. • Dab, whiting ... (16.5%)
30. • Snails (16.3%)
31. • Hake (15.9%)
32. • Marinated Tuna (15%)
33. • Egg whites (11.1%)
34. • Skim milk (3.5%)

This issue forces us to stop at an important food: the eggs. The egg is important for supplementation because is readily available, inexpensive and very rich in protein and, in my own opinion, it is the best natural substitute for the Whey protein. Sometimes it happens that we cannot acquire the whey protein because of its high cost or lack thereof in the market and, then, we do not have another option than interrupt our diet and protein cycle. This really is not necessary if we can consume egg whites. Personally I consider it much more economical, healthy and effective. It is for these reasons that we propose to analyze some properties of the egg protein before moving on to study different types of Whey Protein and its characteristics.

As we said before in this book, eggs are an excellent source of protein. The egg is in the same step of the food pyramid. That mean that one egg is so relevant as meat, poultry, fish, dried beans and nuts. Egg protein is found in the egg all, especially in the white part.

A medium egg (60g) provides about 7 g of protein. These proteins are rich in essential amino acids, and the balance between these amino acids is very good, allowing consider egg protein as a reference protein. In terms of equivalence of food: 2 eggs provide as much protein as 100 g of meat or fish. The energy value of an average egg (60 g) round around 376 kJ (90 kcal). The lipid content is 7 g, which are essentially present in the egg yolk.

2/3 fatty acids are unsaturated; because we must remember that An egg also contains 180 mg of cholesterol. The egg is rich in vitamins A, (100 g of edible part contribute 28.4% of the RDA -CDR-), vitamin D (36%), vitamin E (15.8%), riboflavin (26, 4%), niacin (20.6%), folic (25.6%) acid, vitamin B12 (84%), biotin (40%), pantothenic acid (30%), phosphorus (30.9%), iron (15.7%), zinc (20%) and selenium (18.2%)) and trace elements (iron and zinc).[52] Scott Diedrichs from the Bodybuilding website suggests eat six egg whites and two buds each morning. We can also distribute egg intake throughout the day; so we have to eat many other foods rich in protein during the day in addition to eggs, to achieve our goals.[53] Most bodybuilders should consume 1.5 g of protein per pound of body weight. For example, a 200 pound bodybuilder should consume 300 g of protein per day. We must prepare eggs properly to not get sick. If we eat raw eggs, we will be risking

---

[52] European food information council. Obtenible en http://www.eufic.org/page/es/page/faq/faqid/eggs-nutritional-value/
[53] Are eggs important for bodybuilding ?. Obtainable in http://www.livestrong.com/es/son-buenos-huevos-info_26981/. Consulted on January 3, 2015 at 13: 58hrs.

to infect us with salmonella; but we can avoid this danger when we cook eggs as scrambled, boiled, fried, baked or steamed. It is also important do not eat many eggs per day because the fat and cholesterol that they have can be harmful when you eat too much. Egg whites contain unsaturated fats, and the yolks contain saturated fats, but you can limit your intake of cholesterol if you eat more egg whites than yolks (experts recommend only to consume 2 egg yolks per day). In my personal experience I usually consume 6 whites of eggs daily in the morning with two yolks (fried tortilla) and the rest of the protein intake during the day with extra rations of whey protein. Having analyzed the importance of egg protein for bodybuilders we will continue to analyze other necessary food before boarding the whey Protein. We refer to milk and cheese.

In general milk is understood as liquid and white substance secreted from the breasts of female mammals to feed their young and consists of casein, lactose, inorganic salts, suspended globules of fat and other substances. The most important of all milks is produced by cows, which serves as food and from also we can make cheese, yogurt, butter and other derivatives.

Cow's milk has an average density of 1.032 g / ml. It is a complex and heterogeneous mixture comprising a colloidal system of three phases:

- Solution: minerals and carbohydrates are dissolved in water.
- Suspension: protein substances are suspended with water.
- Emulsion: fat in water is presented as emulsion.

It contains a significant proportion of water (about 87%). The rest constitutes the dry extract represents 130 grams (g) per unit and in which there are 35 to 45 g of fat.

Other main components are lactose carbohydrates, proteins and lipids. The organic components are carbohydrates, lipids, proteins, vitamins, and minerals components are Ca, Na, K,

Mg and Cl. Milk also contains different groups of nutrients. Organic substances (carbohydrates, lipids, proteins) are present in roughly equal amounts and constitute the main source of energy. These nutrients are divided into elements builders, protein, and energetic compounds, carbohydrates and lipids.

The pH of the milk is slightly acidic (pH between 6.6 and 6.8). Another important chemical property is the acidity, or amount of lactic acid contained therein, which is usually around 0.15 to 0.16%. The milk protein substances are the most important in the chemical aspect. They are classified into two groups: proteins (casein is present in 80% of the total protein, whereas whey proteins do 20%), and enzymes.[54]

From 10 liters of cow's milk can be produced about 1 to 2 kg of cheese (mostly of casein) and an average of 8 to 9 kg of whey. Whey is the set

---

[54] BUSHILL, J.H. Y WRIGHT, W.B.: 1964. *Some physical methods of assessing the effects of processing on the structure and properties of milk*, J. Soc. Dayry Technol., 17:3

of all milk components that are not integrated into the coagulation of casein, and according to the type of milk (according to the species from which it came) may have two types of whey, classified by their taste:

- The sweet whey: comes from cheeses coagulated with rennin. Most of this serum is composed of non-protein nitrogen (22% of total) and has a large concentration of lactose (about 4.9% of the serum); It is the richest in protein (0.8%) but very poor in a matter of lactic acid (0.15%). The rest of the serum is a set of salts, minerals and fats that vary from species to species. The pH is between 6 and 6.2.

- The acid whey: comes from cheeses coagulated with acetic acid and is the common product that remains after manufacturing curd and white cheese. Due to low pH (4.6) is corrosive to metals and contains a higher proportion of non-protein nitrogen (27% of total) and has less lactose in concentration (4.3%). This is because it comes from acid milks and therefore, part of the lactose is converted to lactic acid by fermentation, for that reason has more of lactic acid (0.75%). Due to denaturation, it is poorer protein (0.6%). Usually has lower concentration of salts, minerals, and fats and because of this can vary from species to species.

Lactates and phosphates (very common salts in whey): They help keep the acid-base balance and greatly influence the properties of whey (stability and thermal precipitation).[55] The whey has a low proportion of protein, however they have more nutritional quality than caseins from cheese. Excessive production of whey to make cheese has always been a concern and have devised many ways to use it. One of the easiest ways to use buttermilk, homemade type, is heated to precipitate proteins and then press it or to filter it. In many places in Mexico people prefer to eat the

[55] HILL, A.R., IRVINE, D.M.Y BULLOCK, D.H.: (1985). *Buffer capacity of cheese wheys*. J. Food Sci. pp. 50:733.

whey immediately after salting (and called cottage cheese). The industrial applications of whey usually come once it is dehydrated, when is poorly soluble. During evaporation (to remove water) and spray (for drying) it may lose its nutritional properties reason why the pH and temperature of these two processes should be monitored carefully during drying the extract.[56]

Whey proteins are compact, globular, having a molecular weight ranging between 14,000 and 1,000,000 daltons, and are soluble in a wide pH range (remain intact when milk is naturally short, since there has been no presence of heat that denature proteins). In its natural state the whey proteins are not associated with caseins, but in the heat treated and homogenized milk, some of these proteins can be gotten.[57] Whey proteins comprise at least 8 different fractions, all sensitive to high temperatures (thermal processes) and are

---

[56] MATHUR, BN. Y SHAHANI, K.M.: (1979). *Use of total whey constituetens for human food.* J. Dayri Sci. pp. 62:1.

[57] DARGAL BADUI, SALVADOR: (2006). *Química de los Alimentos. Cap. 12 Leche.* Edit. Pearson, Addison Weasley. 4° Edición. p. 614.

therefore the first to degrade in processes such as pasteurization or UHT. The reason that milk is not decomposed when it is out of refrigeration (after being heat treated) is because when whey protein is denatured releases a sulfhydryl group and reduces partially oxidation activity.[58] Whey proteins with greater importance in milk are:

A) α-lactalbumin: the enzyme system is required for the synthesis of lactose. Animal milks do not have this protein does not contain lactose. This protein has no free sulfhydryls but has four disulfides who give the cysteine, which is 2.5 times more sulfur than casein. It has low molecular weight and a high level of tryptophan. It is considered that since a long time ago, birds and cattle were united by a (not taxonomic) genetic common trunk because the amino acid sequence of this protein is similar to egg lysozyme.[59] As a curiosity we can say that this protein is denatured at 63 degrees of temperature.

---

[58] Ibidem.

[59] BREW, K Y GROBLER, J.A.: (1992). *α-Lactalbumin*. Advanced Dairy Chemestry. proteins, vol. 1. Ed. P.F. Fox. pp. 191–229.

B) β-lactoglobulin: it is an insoluble protein in distilled water, but is soluble in dilutions of salts, also is denatured and is precipitated within 73°C (not withstand pasteurization). This protein is not found in human milk, but it is abundant in ruminant, is also considered responsible for some allergic reactions in infants.[60] There are industrial processes that modify the components of cow's milk to make it more similar to human milk and thus be able to give to babies. In these processes this protein fraction is removed by precipitation with polyphosphates or by gel filtration, then is mixed with other components (casein, soybean oil, minerals, vitamins, lysozyme, etc.).[61]

---

[60] WHARTON, B.: (1981). *Inmunological implications of alternatives to mother's milk.* The Inmunology of Infant Feeding. A. Wilkinson, Plenum Press, Nueva York.
[61] AL-MASHIKH, S.A. Y NAKAI, S.: (1987). *Reduction of beta-lactoglobulin content of cheese whey by polyphosphate precipitation.* J. Food Sci. pp. 52:1237; KUWATA, T., PHAN A.M., MA, C.Y. Y NAKAI, S.: (1985). *Elimination of β-lactoglobulin from whey to simulate human milk protein.* J. Food Sci. pp. 50:602; SHAHANI, K.M.: (1979). *Humanized milk.* J. Dairy Sci. Technol. pp. 14:2.; DARGAL BADUI, SALVADOR: (2006). *Química de los Alimentos. Cap. 12 Leche.* Edit. Pearson, Addison Weasley. 4° Edición. p. 614.

C) Whey acidic protein: this protein is a component of milk found only in the category Glires, which groups rodents and lagomorphs, although related sequences have been found in pigs because this protein contains similar domains to protease inhibitors, can be observed that its function is protective of the oral mucosal and antimicrobial.[62]

D) Immunoglobulins: these proteins complete around 10% of total whey proteins and derived from animal blood and belong to the types IgA and IgE and plasma cells derived from connective tissue of the breast. Some scientists, as mentioned above, see this as the reason to be of milk, because it transmits some immunity to breeding (mainly the memory of the diseases that the mother has suffered). They are usually very abundant in colostrum (up to 100g / L).

[62] IDOJI Y, WATANABE Y, YAMASHITA A, YAMANISHI K, NISHIGUCHI S, SHIMADA K, YASUNAGA T, YAMANISHI H: (2008). «In silico study of whey-acidic-protein domain containing oral protease inhibitors». International Journal of Molecular Medicine 21 (4).

Raw milk would not be suitable for marketing and consumption without being subjected to certain industrial processes that would ensure that the microbiological load is within safe limits.[63] Therefore, a milk with health guarantees must have been milked with modern and hygienic methods of suction in which there is no physical contact with milk. After milking, it is cooled and stored in a milk tank and, finally, is transported in isothermal tanks to processing plants. In these plants, milk must be evaluated before discharge to see if it meets with optimal characteristics for consumption.

Among the analysis are the physicochemical analysis (to evaluate the composition of milk fat) and dry extract (among other parameters) to detect possible fraud watered down. The organoleptic assessments are another type of evaluation to the detection of unusual flavors. Finally there are bacteriological tests for the detection of pathogenic bacteria. Thus, Milk that

---

[63] HARPER, J.W. (1976). Processing-induced changes. Dairy Technology and Engineering, The Avi Publishing, Westport, Conn. pp. Psráfrasis the central idea of the book.

does not meet quality requirements, must be rejected. Once verified its optimal state is stored in tanks of large capacity for commercial packaging.

Depuration

Milk, according to the commercial application that will have, can go through a lot of processes known as purification processes. These ensure the sanitary quality of milk, and are listed below:[64]

- Filtering: this process is used to separate the whey protein and thus remove impurities such as blood, hair, straw, manure. For this process a filter or grid is used.
- Homogenization: this physical process involves the continuous agitation (pneumatic or mechanical) with a pump or a homogenizer. The purpose of the homogenization of milk is decreasing fat globule before heating and avoid the cream

---

[64] Ciberhabitat.gob.mx. "Computers in the production of milk powder. '. Archived from the original on 29 November 2015. Accessed April 18, 2008.

forming. This should be 1 micrometer in diameter. When the milk is standardized and fat from milk is regulated, it is mixed with homogenization, preventing further phase separation. It is for these reasons that this process is carried out at 50 ° C to avoid denaturation. The homogenization after pasteurization, stabilizes the fat in small particles that prevent creaming during fermentation and produces a better texture since the interaction between casein and fat globules becomes favorable to dairy products that require fermentation.[65]

- Standardization: when the fat content of the milk does not have the quality required to make specific product is used milk powder or vegetable fat. It is done in two ways: first, mathematically (with procedures like Pearson's x^2 test or material balance) and the other form is the practice, measuring

[65] CHANDAN, R.D., Y SHAHARI, K.M.: (1992). *Yogurt. Cap. 1.* Dairy Science and Technology Handbook, vol. 2. VCH Publishers Inc., NY. pp. 1–56.

the masses and mixing them all. Milk should have 3.5% fat before moving to any process. This process is also used when the milk, heat-treated once, lost some kind of components, which usually happen more in milk with slow levels of calcium and with reincorporated new nutrients.

- Deodorization: used to remove odors that could impregnate milk during their obtaining (dung, for example). This requires a vacuum chamber, where the odors are completely removed. The milk should smell sweet or sour.

- Bactofugation: eliminates bacteria by centrifugation through a machine called bactófuga. In this process, because of a centrifugal rotation, bacterias die and are separated from milk. Finally the Milk should be 300,000 CFU / mL (colony forming units per milliliter). Before making a bactofugation should make an evaluation of bacteria in milk and identify them, this is very important as it allows to determine the most effective method for removing a specific bacteria. It is usually taken as standard that 1800 seconds heating to 80 ° C eliminates the coliforms, the TB bacillus and spores; and inhibition of enzymes alkaline phosphatase and peroxidase. But this is only a highly variable standard that depends on many conditions.

- Clarification: is used to separate solids and unnecessary sediments in milk (like dust or dirt, very small particles that cannot be filtered). Instrument used in this process is called clarifier, but the most important is to know that process can be performed in two ways: heating the milk to 95 ° C and letting it stir for 15 minutes or heating at 120 ° C for 5 minutes.

After the cleansing, milk can be processed for human consumption by heating over low heat for partial or complete removal of bacteria. According to the required target, will be used thermization, pasteurization, ultra-pasteurization or sterilization.

- Termización: This procedure is intended to reduce or inhibit enzyme activity.
- Pasteurization: (Slow High Temperature, SHT): with this procedure milk is heated to certain temperatures for the elimination of specific pathogens: mainly known as Streptococcus thermophilus. Anyway this process also inhibits some other bacteria.
- Ultra-pasteurization: (Ultra High Temperature, UHT): In this procedure is used a higher temperature than pasteurization. Eliminates all existent bacteria but the only exception is the lactic acid bacteria. It requires no further cooling.
- Sterilization: the used high temperature (140 ° C for 45 s) eliminates any microorganisms present in milk. It is not subsequently cooled; this milk is also called sanitized. This process does not apply to flavored milks or reformulated because it could become candy.

- Sterilization: can occur in an autoclaves online called Barriquands. The milk treated in this way are packed in carton boxes or special cardboard sanitized and internally coated with a glossy film.
- Cooling may be dispensable after heat treatment because it is not necessary to lower the temperature in all cases, only when the milk still has microorganisms.

According to the outgoing microbial quality could be considered the possibility of refrigeration or not; hence the thermisation requires cooling and the sterilized process not. Milk will not be altered at room temperature if there is not any bacteria or enzyme activity; but if we leave any milk in a glass and without covering then oxygen will do the same as the oxidizing agent, but not because of internal activities of milk.[66]

---

[66] HEGSTED, MARK (1986). *««Calcium and osteoporosis»»*. *Journal of Nutrition* (116): 2316–2319.

All ideas explained in this book regarding the purification of milk express all trust that we can have in industrial dairy. For all those who regularly attend the gym, milk is essential and its benefits include:

- It contains good amount of calcium: 3 glasses of 200 cc provides up to 800 mg of calcium, covering the minimum requirements and helps to control the overweight. Prevents also the peripheral insulin resistance. Therefore we recommend that when you choose to drink milk take skim milk.

- Provides the body with magnesium, phosphorus and vitamins A, B2, B12 and D; generally favorable for those who train hard.

- Helps bone formation and preventing osteoporosis.

- Reduces levels of uric acid.

- Replaces saliva, neutralizes oral acids, re-mineralize the teeth and prevents cavities.

- It has conjugated with fatty acids (CLA), which enhances immune function and in some way prevents cancers.

- Regulates blood pressure in certain circumstances.

- And also it contains stearic acid which controls blood lipids.

Well, we know that drinking milk is highly recommended ... but when we choose the product begin the doubts in our minds. Do not worry, the semi-skimmed milk is ideal in most cases, but if you have serious problems about gain weight, drink whole milk is the best option. Whole milk is recommended for weight gain because in one liter of whole milk we get 30 grams of fat and more than 600 calories. If you want to lose weight, take skimmed milk will be better.

Whey Protein. Features and varieties.[67]

The whey protein is composed mainly of globular proteins of high biological value extracted from

---

[67] The issue relating to whey in this book has been based mainly in the article "whey protein" of the free encyclopedia Wikipedia. All text has been corroborated with the literature cited in the footnotes and corrected and confirmed by specialists.

whey (one resulting liquid milk as a byproduct during the manufacture of some cheeses). Is generally marketed and used as a dietary supplement for sport activity, especially in order to develop strength or increase muscle mass, because of the main role that proteins play in the muscle resynthesize process.

In addition, experts have attributed, to the whey protein, some beneficial health properties, without conclusive results. Some preclinical studies in rodents have suggested that whey protein may possess anti-cancer properties or anti-inflammatory; however, human data are scarce.[68] The effects of whey protein on human health are of great interest and are being investigated as a way to reduce the risk of disease as well as

[68] HAKKAK R, KOROURIAN S, RONIS MJ, JOHNSTON JM, BADGER TM: (May de 2001). «Dietary whey protein protects against azoxymethane-induced colon tumors in male rats». Cancer Epidemiol. Biomarkers Prev. 10 (5): 555–8; XIAO R, CARTER JA, LINZ AL, FERGUSON M, BADGER TM, SIMMEN FA (September de 2006). «Dietary whey protein lowers serum C-peptide concentration and duodenal SREBP-1c mRNA abundance, and reduces occurrence of duodenal tumors and colon aberrant crypt foci in azoxymethane-treated male rats». J. Nutr. Biochem. 17 (9): 626–34.

possible complementary treatment for various diseases. Although whey protein is responsible for some milk allergies, the major allergen in milk is casein.[69] The whey is obtained when milk coagulates during cheese production, and contains all the soluble milk components after the pH is lowered to 4.6 during the coagulation process.[70] Then, the whey is simply a 5% solution of lactose in water, with some minerals and lactalbumin.[71] In this procedure the fat is removed and then processed for human consumption. The processing can be performed by simply drying or the protein content can be increased by removing lipids and other non-proteinaceous materials.[72] For example, spray drying after membrane filtration is used to separate whey proteins.

---

[69] WAL JM: (November de 2004). «Bovine milk allergenicity». Ann. Allergy Asthma Immunol. **93** (5 Suppl 3): S2–11. BURKS W, HELM R, STANLEY S, BANNON GA: (June de 2001). «Food allergens». Curr Opin Allergy Clin Immunol **1** (3): 243–8

[70] Whey." The Encyclopædia Britannica. 15th ed. 1994

[71] Ibidem.

[72] FOEGEDING, EA; DAVIS, JP; DOUCET, D; MCGUFFEY, MK: (2002). «Advances in modifying and understanding whey protein functionality». Trends in Food Science & Technology **13** (5): 151–9.

The whey can be denatured by high temperatures, especially when we raise the temperature above 72 ° C. However when this does not happen the whey protein that has not been added to the setting process or acidification of milk, makes hydrophobic interactions with other proteins and form a protein gel. [73] However, denatured whey can still cause allergies in some people. [74]

The whey protein is very popular among athletes practitioners of bodybuilding and is mainly used in the ergogenic diet of the sport with the aim of promoting metabolism reactions associated with muscle hypertrophy (muscle growth). The whey protein is sold in the form of soluble powder and must be consumed as milkshakes with certain flavors. The amount of powdered whey protein to consume is adjusted to the nutritional needs of each athlete and his objectives. In some cases the 50% protein that we drink comes from whey

---

[73] Ibidem.
[74] LEE YH: (November 1992). *«Food-processing approaches to altering allergenic potential of milk-based formula.».* J. Pediatr. **121** (5 Pt 2): S47–50.

protein. The powdered concentrates are usually low in fat and cholesterol, making them ideal as complements to other low-fat diets.[75]

The whey protein typically comes in three major forms: concentrate, isolate and hydrolysate).

- Concentrates typically have a low (but still significant) level of fat and cholesterol but generally, compared to other forms of whey protein, have higher levels of bioactive compounds, and carbohydrates in the form of lactose - they contain 29-89% protein by weight. Whey protein concentrated milk (WPC), specifically, is the cheapest and most common form of whey protein and is often used to introduce a larger amount of protein in the diet with the intention of maximizing muscle hypertrophy. Although the protein isolate is made usually by over 90% pure protein, the concentrate reaches at most 89%. This difference is due to the

---

[75] SHAWN M. TALBOTT: *"A Guide to Understanding Dietary Supplements",*

concentrated whey protein contains more carbohydrates (in the form of lactose) and calories than isolation, but this difference does not prevent that many shakes or meal replacements employ these two formulas together. Despite this lower level of concentration, it remains a good quality protein (especially for those who are not lactose intolerant) because the concentrated milk whey includes a generous amount of essential amino acids. It is recommended to consume with breakfast or after training. [76]

- isolates are processed to remove the fat and lactose, but are generally lower in bioactive compounds and contain 90% or more protein by weight. Isolate whey protein has a slight milk flavor.

---

[76] Taken concentrated whey protein hydrolyzate VS VS isolated. Prozis official blog published on May 7th, 2013. available in http://www.prozis.com/blog/es/whey-concentrado-aislado-hidrolizado/. Retrieved January 3, 2015.

(Whey Protein Isolate - WPI) is the purest form of whey protein and is composed of 90% pure protein. This supplement is obtained by filtering the milk protein enough to be practically free of lactose, carbohydrates, fats and cholesterol. It is considered a complete protein, which means it has all the necessary amino acids to the diet, with particularly high levels of BCAA. Another interesting fact is the high level of leucine contained and promotes muscle protein synthesis (and therefore muscle growth), which in turn improves fat loss by the energy that the body needs to perform this process . Whey isolate also contains a lot of cysteine. Women with high levels of cysteine have less risk of breast cancer compared with those with lower levels of cysteine. In addition, pregnant women who obviously need more protein, isolated whey offers an excellent protein source. At elderly people it is also a great help because this form of whey can help prevent bone and muscle degradation.

Because of cost, whey isolate is especially aimed at people with a sensitive digestive system, who have trouble digesting lactose or who are simply demanding and looking for a high quality product with a very small amount of carbohydrates. This kind of protein can be very useful at the end of a drying phase (definition), to decrease the useless dose of carbohydrates from the diet plan.[77] If the isolated protein is presented, in many respects superior to the concentrated protein, it is also true that "purity" has its costs. Thus, although the concentration of pure protein is lower in the concentrated whey, to maintain a good biological value and be more economical, often it becomes the first choice of many athletes. On the other hand, the most exigent athletes or lactose intolerant people prefer protein isolate despite having a higher price, but others give more importance to the rapid uptake of the protein hydrolyzed, which allows better

---

[77] Ibidem.

performance in training and he is responsible for the reputation of "standard formula" that this protein has.

- hydrolysates whey protein are made from proteins that are predigested and partially hydrolyzed in order to make them easier to metabolize, but their cost is generally higher.[78] Highly hydrolysed whey may be less allergenic than other forms of whey.[79]

Whey protein hydrolysate (WPH) is considered as the standard whey protein formula. This protein is enzymatically broken in large peptides, completely different to the process of the concentrated or isolated whey protein. This breaking of the hydrolyzed protein provides a high rate of absorption, making it far above that in terms of improving muscle hypertrophy post training. A protein hydrolyzed supplementation can help stimulate and

---

[78] FOEGEDING, EA; DAVIS, JP; DOUCET, D; MCGUFFEY, MK (2002).: *Ob.cit.*
[79] LEE YH (November 1992): ob.cit.

boost the immune system by increasing the level of glutathione, which helps detoxify the body and protect cells of the immune system. Because the added value of the hydrolyzed whey protein is rapidly assimilated, we can assume that this is the best protein to take immediately after training. Hydrolyzed proteins generally have very bad taste, so here are some tips to consider when you're buying a product of hydrolyzed whey:[80]

1- The product should indicate the degree of hydrolysis applied to the protein. The higher percentage of hydrolysis means that the flavor is more bitter. If the product does not offer this detail, ask the manufacturer.

2- The label should display a table with the molecular weights of the peptides. These are measured in Dalton. Usually the percentage of the peptides are listed, for example, MW 20,000-40,000 Dalton 40%.

---

[80] Ibidem

3- WPH contain virtually no fractions of biologically active proteins. All fractions are destroyed during the process.

4- If you see any demand greater than 104 BV, you must be careful because this is not possible.

In theory WPH is ideal to drink immediately after workout because your body will absorb it very quickly. This simply happens because it is more available (pre-digested) than other whey. As there is still oligopeptides chains, the body will use both methods of protein absorption in the intestine. However, the fact that there is not fractions of biologically active proteins could be seen as a drawback of this WPH. So for this reason, you should use hydrolyzed whey protein in the intra-workout or pre and post workout, using other types of whey at other times of day.[81]

---

[81] Ibidem.

Shakes of whey protein, addition to providing protein, have also been linked to increasing insulin levels in the blood. The whey increases insulin secretion from beta cells in the pancreas; so it is important to have in mind that insulin is an anabolic hormone and participates in the metabolism of carbohydrates, also pushes glucose into muscle cells, and also helps the use of muscle protein. Hence when we consume shake of whey protein, not only we are helping to increase the amount of protein available for muscle cells because they are also helping the renewal mechanism's own muscle cells. The hydrolyzed (WPH) has been proven very effective to increase the maximum concentration of insulin through a mechanism that is not related to gastric emptying (Power et al, 2008). The WPH has essential amino acids that facilitate secretion of insulin beta cells. Whey protein is composed of 40-50% and EAAs is considered a rich source of insulin to regulate the absorption of these amino acids to make them more bioavailable. The key amino acids for this is thought to be "phenylalanine" although the exact mechanism is not fully understood.[82]

How you should drink Whey protein?

People who regularly attend the gym and are supplemented with Whey Protein do it for two purposes: to gain muscle mass or burn fat. First we must be clear and be aware that whey protein supplementation is indicated for athletes who train with median / high intensity and are not able to recover or increase their muscle mass with oral well adapted and personalized diet. Bodybuilding, athletics, weightlifting, are the disciplines in which this protein supplementation is more appropriate.

accurately determine the best program for the consumption of whey protein depends on each person and specifically varies depending on the diet, sex and age time. However, there are three key moments to ensure greater effectiveness by consuming this protein:

---

[82] Ibidem.

When you wake up in the morning: the whey protein can also be consumed early in the morning because at that time, as a result of the sleep period, the levels of protein in our body have decreased.

Immediately after training: Another of the most suitable moments for the consumption of whey protein supplements seems to be immediately after physical exercise moments. At this point it is when the muscles of athletes have suffered, and are more susceptible to incorporate new components to its structure. There are authors who believe that the fractional making this protein throughout the day improves its effectiveness by depositing more staggered into the muscle, though they agree that one of the doses made after the exercise to get muscle recovery can work more effectively.

A half hour before bedtime: take whey protein before bedtime helps reduce protein degradation that is caused naturally during our sleep time. In this sense, if we want to increase muscle mass, whey protein consumed at this time will help to avoid this degradation during our off hours. Although, on the contrary, if our primary objective is the development and construction of muscle protein degradation that occurs during sleep could be favorable.

However, we must never forget that this is a supplement and is encompassed within a daily diet and an intense sports activity. By this we mean that it is possible that all the nutrients needed for the perfect sport and the best possible performance from normal diet is already obtained. Only when this does not happen is when taking this supplement may be recommended. To find out if whey protein consumption is necessary or not, you should consult with a healthcare professional to assess the requirements and diet. When a person follows a regular diet should only take whey protein if the specialist recommends it for him. Calculating how much to take is individual and is associated with many factors that need to be studied.

There is no uniform rule regarding the amount of whey protein that we must take daily because it depends on many factors. Most experts recommend consuming at least 1 g of whey protein per kilogram of weight and not more than 1.8g / kg. Other specialists prefer the called "rule of 30g" which stipulates that people should consume 30g of whey protein as a standard dose for each supplementation. Anyway, whey protein packages always announce the amount of services they have and bring a spoon (25-30 g) as a means of measurement. This way is much easier for the athlete to apply the rule of 30g. Finally I note that when we talk about the amount of grams of protein that should be consumed in one day we refer to the total quantity of all meals. So if you consume eggs, meat, milk and whey protein during the day should keep in mind the amount of protein that you are adding to your body. The first sign that you are consuming more protein is the appearance of pimples all over the skin, headaches and sudden stimulation of sexual appetite.

Theme VI: Testosterone

It is an androgen steroid and also the main male sex hormone. In men, testosterone plays a key role in the development of the male reproductive tissues such as the testes and prostate. Testosterone also contributes to promoting secondary sexual characteristics such as increased muscle mass and bone and body hair growth. In addition, testosterone is essential for health and wellness as for the prevention of osteoporosis. On average testosterone concentration in the blood plasma of an adult male is ten times greater than that of women. The daily natural secretion of testosterone in men is 5 to 10 micrograms per liter of blood and women 0.4 mcg.[83]

---

[83] Taken from DOMINGUEZ, EDWARD Total Culturismo blog. Obtainable in http://culturismototal.blogspot.com/2013/02/la-testosterona.html. Retrieved January 3, 2016 at 12: 34hrs.

The body uses cholesterol as a basis for the development of this hormone. These androgens are produced by Leydig cells in the testicles. The amount of synthesized testosterone is regulated by the hypothalamic-pituitary-testicular axis. When testosterone levels are low, the gonadotropin releasing hormone is released by the hypothalamus which in turn stimulates the pituitary gland to release FSH and LH. These last two hormones stimulate the testicles to synthesize testosterone. When we supplement our body with high doses of testosterone, the hypothalamus and the pituitary gland react by a negative feedback to inhibit the release of GnRH and FSH / LH respectively. So when there is an excess consumption of testosterone the first signs manifest with severe headaches in the region of the pituitary gland.

Consuming forms of testosterone are two: by intramuscular injection or by oral consumption. When it is supplemented by the injection, it enters directly into the bloodstream, but when it is consumed by tablet reaches the liver via the gastrointestinal tract, here the substance is partially destroyed and sent to the bloodstream in their original form. In this way increases production of erythropoiesis stimulating factors and, consequently, erythrocytes increase. The testosterone is related in 90% with the protein when it enters in the body and its quickest route of assimilation is intravenous way. we should also note that the testosterone is eliminated from the body by the kidneys.[84] Therefore it is recommended that during the period of its supplementation we consume at least a half-liter of water daily.

Therapy Testosterone replacement is used in cases of male hypogonadism, suppression of lactation, breast carcinoma hormone-dependent advanced endometriosis, menopause associated with estrogen, frigidity, Aplastic Anemia, Osteoporosis with gonadal deficiency, Phase oligoanuria of I.R. acute. Treatment of hypoactive sexual desire disorder in bilaterally ovariectomized and hysterectomized women. For

---

[84] Ibidem.

bodybuilders, testosterones generally produce large increases in mass muscle and strength, but they tend to have more side effects and loss of muscle mass at the end of therapy if not completed the cycle in the correct way. Supplementation with testosterone also causes a large water retention, and this should be very taken into account, especially in periods of definition. Testosterone is the base of the pyramid of all well-structured cycles.

Testosterone administration generally should not be more than 8 weeks. We recommend lengthen the cycle between 2 or 4 weeks with only anabolic compounds. In this way, we ensure that the recovery of self-testosterone production in the body be effective, because, conversely, if the cycle is prolonged, side effects will be negative. Testosterone supplementation get effect on our body between 2 and 3 weeks, it is for these reasons that we recommend that the cycle last a minimum of six weeks. Testosterone also causes baldness strongly and it is very important to consider, especially for bodybuilders older than 33 years old because the enzyme 5-alpha-reductase converts testosterone into dihydrotestosterone (DHT) which is responsible for atrophy of hair follicles, causing consequently, scalp membranes and making hair be more rigid. During this process Follicular structure is saturated and receives less blood supply and new hairs are born weaker and thinner than normal and with a bad healthy. As a result, atrophied follicles and fallen hair will never be replaced.[85]

How to consume testosterone?

As we said earlier, there are two ways to consume testosterone: intravenously (injection) or orally (capsules, tablets). Many times people inject in body large amounts of testosterone into thinking that soon they will obtain greater results in shortest period of time. This is completely wrong and foolish. The therapeutic guidelines recommend that one bodybuilder should receive injections between 100 to 250 mg every 3-4 weeks or between 250- 500 mg per week, being

---

[85] Ibidem.

able to reach the 750 mg in bodybuilders over 100 kilos. However we recommend that you consult a doctor or specialist on the topic before starting a cycle because testosterone supplementation abuse can lead to hypersensitivity; prostate cancer or breast cancer in man; presence or history of liver cancer, renal dysfunction, liver disease, hypertension, heart failure, hypercalcemia, edema, hypoproteinemia, benign prostatic hypertrophy, epilepsy, migraine, diabetes mellitus, xerostomia, may potentiate sleep apnea in patients with obesity and chronic respiratory disease, liver failure. Concomitant use with warfarin increases anticoagulant effect and increases the concentration of cyclosporine, oxyphenbutazone and decreases blood glucose concentration. It also decreases the level of TBG, make to the person more aggressive, raises cholesterol, shrinking of the testicles, among other effects.[86]

Testosterone is totally contraindicated in people with liver tumors, kidney failure or pregnant

---

[86] Ibidem.

women. Some of the adverse reactions consumption testosterone are Polycythemia, weight gain, hot flashes, acne, baldness, increased prostate specific antigen, abnormal test prostate, benign prostatic hyperplasia, reactions in the injection site, diarrhea, hypertension ; dizziness, paresthesia, amnesia, hyperesthesia, mood disorders; prostatic disorders, gynecomastia, breast pain, headache; hypercholesterolemia, hypertriglyceridemia, hyperlipidemia; depression at the end of the cycle, headache, liver damage and kidney. However we stress that all these negative effects can be avoided if the testosterone is supplemented in the amounts indicated in this book; especially if it will be applied intravenously. In the case that the testosterone be supplemented orally, we recommend following the instructions of the container. It is generally recommended to consume between 2 or 4 pills daily. It depends on the pharmaceutical product characteristics. This last recommendation is very important because many people believe that by stopping the cycle or intensifying activity in the gym will eliminate these adverse effects and finally culminate worsening their situation. That is why we reiterate the necessity to first consult a doctor at all times.

Theme VII: The L-carnitine

In animals, carnitine is synthesized mainly in the liver and kidney from the amino acids lysine (through lysine trimethyl) and methionine. In many proteins, lysine residues can suffer mono-, di- and trimethylation. By hydrolyzing these proteins is created amino acid N6, N6, N6-trimethyl lysine (TML), which is used as precursor in the biosynthesis of carnitine. At the same time, by action of the enzyme trimethyl lysine dioxygenase (TML-DO, EC 1.14.11.8) position 3 of the TML is hydroxylated to form 3-hydroxy-N6, N6-trimethyl lysine (HTML) in the presence of diatomic oxygen as the oxidizing agent , α-ketoglutarate as electron acceptor, in addition to iron (II) and ascorbic acid as cofactors. This is the only reaction takes place in the mitochondria, while the following takes place in the cytosol. The HTML suffers a reverse aldol condensation to form glycine and N4, N4, N4-trimetilaminobutiraldehído

(TMABA) and, In this step, aldolase enzyme lysine hidroxitrimetil (HTMLA, EC 4.1.2. "X") and pyridoxal phosphate as a cofactor are required. After, The aldehyde group is oxidized to become carboxylic acid to form the γ-butyrobetaine (γBB) thanks to the trimetilaminobutiraldehído dehydrogenase (TMABA-DH, EC 1.2.1.47), which requires NAD + as electron acceptor. The γ butyrobetaine is hydroxylated at the 3 position to give final product as carnitine, reaction catalyzed by the enzyme butyrobetaine dioxygenase (γBB-DO, EC 1.14.11.1), requiring iron (II), 3-oxoglutarate, and ascorbic acid as cofactors. As we can see, after a cumbersome process and various chemical reactions is obtained L-carnitine. Hence the first conclusion is that L-carnitine is an amino acid found naturally in our body.

Many are the qualities of the L-carnitine because it is able to give us more energy, lose weight, increase our immune system, stimulate the mental faculties and decreases cholesterol and triglycerides. Carnitine is a nutrient similar to vitamins and is capable of performing all the above and even more. Carnitine as amino acid and its role in biochemical reactions is already well studied. With this we mean that L-carnitine has been studied for many years. Carnitine was discovered early last century, separating the meat extract and determined its chemical structure: beta-hydroxy-gamma acid (tri-methylamino) butyric acid.[87]

Most adults consume about 50 mg of carnitine in their daily nutritional intake. This amount is not enough for optimal health and especially if our sport is bodybuilding. Vegetarians, often, do not eat enough carnitine in their diet because they do not like the meat, and L-carnitine is found primarily in animal foods such as red meat or milk. In these cases and in very specific population groups (elderly, athletes, pregnant women and children.) supplementation with L-carnitine will be absolutely necessary.

Natural sources of L-carnitine include:

---

[87] Taken from Fisiculturismo.es. obtainable in http://www.fisioculturismo.es/fisioculturismo-l-carnitina--estudio-completo.html. Retrieved January 3, 2016 at 2: 09hrs.

- sheep meat: 210 mg / 100 grams
- Lamb: 78 mg / 100 grams
- Veal: 64 mg / 100 grams
- Chicken: 7.5 mg / 100 grams
- Yeast: 2 , 4 mg / 100g
- Milk 2.0 mg / 100 g
- Wheatgerm: 1.0 mg / 100g
- Peanuts: 0.1 mg / 100g
- Cauliflower: 0.1 mg / 100g

Symptoms of deficiency of L-carnitine in the body are:

- Symptoms of deficiency of L-carnitine deposits fats (triglycerides) in the tissues.
- Fatty degeneration of the heart tissue, liver, muscle (lipidosis).
- Fatigue and loss of vitality.
- Muscle atrophy, fatigue.
- Increased recovery time. Immune system depression.
- Deterioration of blood parameters (hematocrit, hemaglobina, etc).

- Decreased sperm activity; infertility.
- Growth disorders in children.
- Cardiovascular disorders: heart failure, angina, arrhythmia.
- Liver disorders: cirrhosis, liver disturbances. Reduction in protein synthesis.
- Increased susceptibility to toxic metabolites free radicals such as ammonium or radicals.

Among the metabolic functions of the carnitine are:

- L-Carnitine is essential for the transport of fatty acids to long mitochondria cell to be converted into energy chain
- Increases beta oxidation of fat.
- It is necessary for the contribution and energy production.
- Helps cellular detoxification, expelling the toxic concentration of acetyl coenzyme A and regulating blood concentrations of ammonia.
- Promotes cellular metabolism by stimulating output units and acetyl acyl groups out of mitochondria.

- It is stored as acetyl or acyl carnitine is an energy source quick release.
- Protects the cell membrane against destruction by free radicals, help cells recover from radical damage. For example, it has been shown to accelerate the speed that the cell repair damaged DNA.
- Increases protein synthesis.
- Promotes the synthesis of Acetylcholine is a brain neurotransmitter from the Hill.
- Increases all metabolic processes involved in the acetil CoA well as the metabolism of glucose and protein metabolism. There is a strong correlation between carnitine and the Krebs cycle and the glycolytic pathway.
- Carnitine stimulates the activity of the enzyme pyruvate dehydrogenase.

Function of L-carnitine in athletic performance I:

The effect of L-carnitine on exercise has been studied in both animals and humans. All evidence shows that L-carnitine increases athletic performance and improves both aerobic and anaerobic capacity.

- Taken before training, the L-carnitine gets:
- Raise submaximal exercise performance
- Increase the maximum aerobic power.
- Promoting savings in liver and muscle glycogen during high intensity exercise and very long.
- Improve glucose utilization in anaerobic exercises
- Increase energy production in sprinters
- Increase VO2 max up to 6% -11%
- Increase the resistance and final effort, avoiding the appearance of "bumps" after 70-90 minutes of intake
- Reduce the production of lactic acid (muscle soreness)

Function of L-carnitine in athletic performance II:

- The L-carnitine achieved a drastic reduction of muscle pain.
- Reduction of ammonium radicals produced by metabolism after intense physical exertion. By reducing the production of ammonia, detoxification increases.

- Increases muscle performance especially in untrained individuals
- Less prone to micro-lesions and infections (stimulates the immune system)
- Helps stabilize the psyche even under stress or intense training phases.
- Reduced recovery time.
- Increases vitality.
- Reduces the heart rate during exercise, so the heart does the same effort with minor heartbeat

Function of L-carnitine in athletic performance III:

- Reduces stress enzyme release
- Prevents loss of L-carnitine, typical of sports long term.
- Intensify the effect of muscle training (not only increases muscle strength but increases the definition and muscle growth)
- Increases circulation and respiration as well as improves muscle oxygenation.
- Increases the average life of red blood cells
- Helps prevent myocarditis typical of athletes

- Improves the function of the diaphragm and abdominal breathing

L-carnitine helps prevent the appearance of premature fatigue and mental exhaustion and even lack of energy that usually occurs the day after the workout. This is done for several reasons:
- To increase concentration and mental capacity
- By reducing ammonium radicals
- Because of its positive effect on the nerves and brain
- By stimulating effect of endorphins
- By improving muscle condition (muscle growth, increased strength and definition)

L-carnitine is very beneficial in reducing body weight. It has shown to reduce blood lipid levels and fat levels in various tissues, particularly when they are abnormally high (as is the case of obese individuals); although there are specialists in this regard should not be considered L-carnitine as a fat burner. The truth is that this is a fairly discussed and scattered throughout the literature concerning the subject matter. What is there is no doubt that L-carnitine helps prevent hunger and low-calorie diets typical of fatigue. It also prevents ketosis or overproduction, typical of diets low in carbohydrates and calories ketones, and is highly recommended to incorporate into a workout plan, especially aerobic type.

L-carnitine as a stimulant of the immune function:
- Carnitine produces a stimulation of the entire immune system
- The L-carnitine promotes the functioning of the immune system because it provides macrophages (phagocytic cells) enough to move quickly through the body to eliminate the intruders such as viruses, bacteria or fungi force.
- To reduce fatigue and increase vitality, the body is less susceptible to disease
- Carnitine provides more energy to fight disease or tumor cells

How to drink L-Carnitine:

- The recommended dose of carnitine supplements are 15 to 30 mg per kilogram of body weight per day.

- The most appropriate for taking L-carnitine time is half an hour before training.

- According to all investigations conducted so far, there is no known negative interaction with any medication. And only under certain circumstances may occur a decrease in the absorption of L-carnitine when taken together with amino acid supplements or protein shakes high concentration. Therefore, we recommend taking both supplements at different times, to ensure optimum effect.

- It is also not recommended to take L-carnitine with dietary fiber or Chitosan as it could drag and remove the feces.

- This supplement has no side effects at recommended doses. Doses above 3 grams per day, can cause diarrhea in susceptible individuals.

- Not under any circumstances one dopant, on the contrary, it is a completely natural substance, which in fact is in the body to perform many beneficial functions. It is not a medicine.

Presentations of L-carnitine:

L-carnitine as a dietary supplement in the sport, is generally marketed in liquid form or in capsules and tablets for oral intake. The most common presentation in which it is marketed is the tartrate salt of carnitine.

Carnitine appears very frequently in formulas with ingredients that stimulate metabolism, such as inositol, choline, B vitamins, methionine and betaine. Synergy carnitine - vitamin C is also used because ascorbic acid is very important for the synthesis of carnitine in the body and both avoid the appearance of fatigue typical of some population groups (elderly, athletes, etc.)

Acetyl-carnitine (ALC) is a special form of carnitine that has the unique ability to optimize brain function. ALC is capable of crossing the blood-brain barrier more readily than carnitine alone. It is very useful for people over 40 years to stimulate the function of neural cells. Carnitine occurs in two chemical forms: L-carnitine and D-carnitine, whose difference is the spatial structure (levorotatory, dextrorotatory). However, the consequence of this difference is that D-carnitine has a toxic effect as it is able to deplete the L-carnitine. In addition, the D form have none of the benefits of the L (the body synthesizes only L-carnitine).

Theme VIII: Caffeine and multivitamins.

Caffeine is a substance present in many elements of the daily diet, and has stimulating effects. There are conflicting views regarding its use because many of its effects are valuable for everyday life. But it can also produce harmful effects if caffeine is used in excessive doses. As with other drugs, excessive drinking can lead to dependence, albeit with a much more benign withdrawal than in other cases. Symptoms of caffeine are headache, irritability and drowsiness. In general, people turn to it to get stimulation, decreasing tiredness and fatigue. It acts as a stimulant of the central nervous system, helping memory, facilitating the association of ideas and improving sensory perception. Caffeine, in perspective, can increase attention and facilitates the biochemical process that develops during the formation of memory in the brain. The main soda or carbonated drinks contain caffeine.[88]

Excesses

Other effects can be dangerous. It increases blood pressure, promoting urine formation and increases cardiopulmonary activity. High doses of caffeine causes excessive excitement, anxiety and insomnia, tremor, hyperesthesia (exaggerated sensitivity increase) and hyporeflexia (diminution of reflexes). Also it stimulates gastric acid secretion, causing gastric intolerance frequently. Therefore, the use of caffeinated beverages along with ulcerogenic drugs, as the aspirins, is not recommended. The use of caffeine is considered Doping in sport because it improves physical performance and maximum blood concentration of caffeine is reached 30 to 45 minutes after ingestion. As found in many anti-flu preparations in association with other drugs, many of these they are also prohibited in circumstances of sporting

---

[88] Taken from fisiculturismo.es. Accessed January 3, 2016 at 02: 09hrs.

competition. The use of certain drugs with stimulant purposes may in fact have the opposite effect in the long term, because caffeine speeds up the expenditure of metabolic resources. It is investigated for years what kind of changes occur in the structures of brain cells after long supplementation with caffeine.

It has been theorized that dendritic spines, extending from the central body to neurons, keep calcium and this may be expelled to the intercellular space under exposure of the caffeine. It is believed that these calcium deposits play a regulatory role in signal transmission in the brain. Apparently, the release of calcium induced by caffeine causes rapid and significant proliferation of existing dendritic spines in the hippocampus, a key brain region for learning and memory.[89]

As we said earlier, there are many criteria on the effects of caffeine on the human organism. Some are positive and some negative, but the truth is that we are talking about a substance that is

---

[89] Ibidem.

consumed by millions of people around the world, day by day, and in quantities and varied forms. Some scientists believe it is a stimulant capable of producing very difficult addiction to break, and therefore must be classified as a drug. Other experts have concluded that caffeine, consumed moderately, is harmless and even beneficial to the human body because it stimulates many of its vital functions. Like most of the elements of the diet, caffeine and products containing it should be used rationally and without excesses.[90]

Meanwhile, vitamins and minerals are vital for normal growth and development. The body does not produce enough or any organic compounds that need, the rest will come from a balanced diet and supplements occasionally. One thing to understand is that when we do not take the amount of vitamins and minerals required by the body can potentially cause a deficiency in the functioning of that body. The body needs 13 vitamins: A, C, D, E, K and B vitamins (niacin, riboflavin, thiamine, biotin, folic acid, pantothenic

---

[90] Ibidem.

acid, B6 and B12) . Vitamins are classified into two categories: soluble and lip soluble.

Top 10 Vitamins for Bodybuilders[91]

10. Cobalamin (B12)

Although the functions of vitamin B12 are numerous, those most important to bodybuilders include carbohydrate metabolism and maintenance of nervous system tissue (spinal cord and nerves that carry signals from the brain to muscle tissues). Stimulation of muscles via nerves is a critical step in the contraction, so coordination and growth of muscles is an important function of vitamin B12. Vitamin B12 is available only in foods of animal origin; therefore, it is very important for athletes under strict vegetarian diet to consult a physician about vitamin B12 supplementation. In fact, B12 is very popular with athletes, even no vegetarians, many of whom swear it helps them perform better.

---

[91] Vitamins for fitness and bodybuilding. In Musculación.net. Accessed January 4, 2016 at 08: 56hrs.

9. Biotin

Although there is a limited amount of sports nutrition research on Biotin, it is part of our top 10 list because it has important functions in amino acid metabolism and the production of energy from many sources. It can also be a vitamin which some bodybuilders have a problem when attempting to maintain an adequate supply. the cause of the difficulties of bodybuilders to consume Biotin is because it can be blocked by a substance called Avidin. The Avidin is found in raw egg whites, a staple for many athletes. In fact, bodybuilders who eat raw egg whites or who do not cook the egg may very well experience problems of growth, Biotin deficiency if their egg white consumption approaches 20 per day. Eating raw eggs can also lead to a bacterial infection called Salmonella, which can have severe health consequences.

8. Riboflavin (Vitamin B2)

Riboflavin is involved in energy production in three areas: 1) Glucose metabolism, 2) Oxidation of fatty acids, and 3) the coming and going of hydrogen ions through the Krebs cycle. Of particular interest to bodybuilders, Riboflavin is somewhat related to protein metabolism. In fact, there is a strong relationship between lean body mass and dietary riboflavin. A study by Belko and colleagues found that women need higher levels of RDA for Riboflavin to return blood levels of Riboflavin to normal after exercise. Another study by Haralambie showed that Riboflavin supplementation improved the muscular hyperexcitability (seen in trained athletes). This vitamin may prove especially important for athletes.

7. Vitamin A

Most of us know that vitamin A helps with vision, but bodybuilders need become familiar with its other benefits. First, vitamin A is important in protein synthesis, the main process of muscle growth. Second, vitamin A is involved in the production of Glycogen, the storage form of energy in the body to yield high intensity. The problem with vitamin A in bodybuilders is twofold. First, American diets are, consequently, designed to be low in vitamin A. Second, vigorous physical activity (which disrupts the absorption of vitamin A) and a low fat diet (vitamin running a loss in feces) puts in danger level of vitamin A in the body. Athletes and bodybuilders should be careful in the consumption of vitamin A during the preparation of the competition.

6. Vitamin E

Vitamin E is a powerful antioxidant, meaning this is to protect cell membranes. It is important because many of the metabolic processes in the body, including the recovery and growth of muscle cells, are dependent on healthy cell membranes. You've probably heard a lot about antioxidants in the news lately, and researches continues to validate their importance. Specifically, antioxidants help to reduce the number of free radicals in the body. Free radicals are natural byproducts of cellular respiration, but the accumulation of free radicals can lead to cellular changes and destruction cells (even cancer) unable to adapt running normally. This means that a reduction in exercise induced processes in the cell such as repair and growth.

5. Nicotinic acid (vitamin B3)

This vitamin is involved in nearly 60 metabolic processes related to energy production and ranks high for bodybuilders by virtue of its fundamental importance in the fuel supply training (untrained, no gain) The bad news is that they have found high levels of nicotinic acid in the blood of athletes after exercise, suggesting that athletes may need more niacin than non-athletes. Moreover, the good news is that even if a diet is low in Niacin, the body can do the amino acid tryptophan, which is found in abundance in turkey meat. Bodybuilders are familiar with the form of Niacin known as nicotine acid, which causes vasodilation and may help to have a competitor look more vascular before going to a competition. But this form of Niacin should not be used during training; large doses of nicotinic acid (50 -. 100 mg) significantly impair the body's ability to mobilize and burn fat.

4. Vitamin D

Vitamin D plays a crucial role in the absorption of calcium and phosphorus. Calcium is needed for muscle contraction. If adequate calcium deposits are not available in the muscle, contractions with muscular strength cannot be sustained. Of course, Calcium is also necessary for the integrity of bones, which must support increased muscle tissue and provide an anchor during muscle contraction. Phosphorus cannot be forgotten. Phosphorus helps provide quick, powerful muscular contractions, which comprise the majority of movements during weight lifting. Phosphorus is also required for the synthesis of ATP (Adenosine Triphosphate), the high energy molecule used by your muscle cells during contraction. This nutrient is on the list because bodybuilders typically avoid the fat content and forget the phosphorus as a necessary component of supplementation. Therefore we recommend drinking a lot of milk daily.

3. Thiamine (vitamin B1)

This B vitamin packs the muscle. Thiamine is one of the vitamins required for protein metabolism and growth. It is also involved in the formation of hemoglobin, a protein found in red blood cells that carries oxygen throughout the body (especially working muscles). The transport of oxygen is critical to athletic performance and becomes even more important when intensity and duration of exercise increase. To Making matters more interesting, we can say that Thiamine, according to researches, it is one of the few vitamins that enhances performance when it is supplemented and because of that is increasingly coveted by athletes. Thiamine requirements appear to be directly related to caloric expenditure. As more frequent is the exercise intensity and duration increase, the more Thiamine is needed.

2. Vitamin B6 (Pyridoxine)

Protein metabolism, growth and carbohydrate utilization are all possible in part by the presence of vitamin B6. Vitamin B6 is second on the list for a very good reason: This is the only vitamin directly tied to protein intake. While more protein you eat, more Pyridoxine is necessary in your body. Of course, this, coupled with Pyridoxine's role in growth, has profound meanings for bodybuilders, though not generally known or discussed in sports nutrition circles.

1. Vitamin C (Ascorbic Acid)

Most athletes do not understand how the presence of vitamin C in our body guarantee a successful physical body. As the most extensively studied vitamin in sports nutrition, Ascorbic acid has proven itself to be valuable to bodybuilders from many points of view. First, vitamin C is an antioxidant protective of muscle cells and also enhancing the recovery and growth.

Second, Ascorbic acid is also involved with amino acid metabolism, especially the formation of Collagen. Collagen is the primary constituent of connective tissue, the stuff that holds your bones and muscles together. This may not seem important, but when you lift heavier weights, the stress you put on your structure becomes tremendous. If your connective tissue is not as healthy and strong as it should be (one problem often seen in steroid users), the risk of injury increases dramatically.

Third, vitamin C helps in the absorption of iron. Iron is necessary to help catch oxygen to hemoglobin in the blood. Without adequate oxygen transportation in blood, muscles are deprived of precious oxygen and performance is greatly reduced.

Fourth, Ascorbic acid also was in the formation and release of steroid hormones, including the anabolic hormone testosterone.

Finally, vitamin C is perhaps the most water soluble vitamin. In other words, it dissolves very quickly in the water. Because muscle cells are essentially water, when a bodybuilder starts training in the gym vitamin C is dispersed in the muscle in big quantities and, consequently, the concentration of this ground substance is made in the body tissues. Then, vitamin C is greatly coveted by bodybuilders.

Bodybuilders are notorious for overlooking these key components of growth and performance. For these reasons, we recommend that you analyze your diet to ensure that you take enough of the vitamins mentioned in this chapter. Remember: You could have the best diet in the world in terms of calories, fat, etc., but if you lack adequate levels of these metabolic spark plugs, you're doing nothing.

How to consume vitamins?[92]

1- Before you start taking vitamins, it is best to consult with your doctor or pharmacist to ensure that its consumption is not harmful to your health. Note that certain vitamin supplements can have serious side effects if are consumed under certain conditions or with certain health problems, also if vitamins are consumed with other medications. You should go to your doctor, especially if you suffer from some type of chronic illness or are subject to a specific drug treatment.

2 -Carefully follow the instructions and warnings on the packaging of vitamins to avoid taking more than necessary. It is advisable to take the lowest effective dose to avoid side effects or overdose; however, if this occurs, call a doctor immediately to the center control. If you have an adverse or allergic reaction to any vitamins, immediately

---

[92] MARTÍNEZ, MARÍA: How to properly take vitamins? In deportes.uncomo.com. obtainable in http://deporte.uncomo.com/articulo/como-tomar-correctamente-las-vitaminas-802.html. Retrieved January 3, 2016 at 23: 45hrs.

interrupt their consumption and consult your doctor.

3- To that vitamin supplements are effective, you must eat well and not take them on an empty stomach. You must remember at all times that vitamins, in any case, never are substitute of the healthy foods but serve as a supplement to meet the nutritional deficiencies of certain foods. You have to take into account that some vitamins cannot be combined with each other; for example, iron should not be combined with other vitamins or calcium. Thus, it is not advisable to take iron with dairy products that contain calcium, but can take it accompanied by orange juice, very rich in vitamin C and contributes to the absorption.

4- You must be consistent when taking vitamins. It is advisable to have specific periods of time or to take vitamins and avoid skipping days. If you are normally very busy, you can set a reminder for certain times, thereby avoiding forget the consumption time. If you are not constant, the body does not absorb vitamins properly and, therefore, these are not effective and do not help you meet your nutritional deficiencies.

5- Do not take vitamins with drinks cold or very hot, because in that case you will avoid that vitamins dissolve properly when they are ingested. It is recommended that vitamins are digested accompanied by some water and follow the instructions specified in the product packaging in order to avoid possible health problems or adverse reactions.

Theme IX: Omega 3

Omega 3 is a lipid substance belonging to the group of fatty acid (FA) polyunsaturated long chain. These are formed by a carboxyl group and a carbon chain variable length molecules. The most important types of Omega 3 are eicosapentaenoic acid (EPA) and docosahexaenoic acid (DHA). Meanwhile, alpha-linolenic acid (ALA) is a type of Omega 3 present in vegetables. The natural product Omega 3 *Codeco Nutrilife* offers the right amount of Omega 3, effective to benefit the body, regulate cholesterol levels and protect heart health.

Omega 3 is found in fish or deep cold water and shellfish, for example:
• Tuna
• Mackerel
• Sardines
• Salmon
• Trout

- Mussels
- Ostras

It is also found in plant foods such as:

- purslane (whole plant)
- Lettuce (leaf)
- Soy (seed)
- Spinach (plant)
- Strawberries (fruit)
- Cucumber (fruit)
- Brussels sprouts (leaves)
- Coles (leaves)
- Pineapple (fruit)
- Almonds
- Nuts

There are natural supplements that contain Omega 3 extracted from fish oil. Such is the case of Omega 3 Codeco Nutrilife, which also contains vitamin E to prevent fatty acids (EPA) and (DHA) rust.

Some of the benefits of Omega 3 are:

• Reduces levels of triglycerides and cholesterol

• prevents the formation of clots in the arteries by preventing platelet aggregation

• Lowers blood pressure in people with mild hypertension

• thin the blood and protects the body from heart attacks, strokes, stroke, angina pectoris, Raynaud's disease, etc.

• Increases power transmissions heart that regulates the heart rate and prevent cardiovascular disease

• Protects against cancer, especially colon cancer, prostate and breast

• It has anti-inflammatory function and relieves pain of diseases such as rheumatoid arthritis and Crohn's disease.

• Promotes the formation of cell membranes

• Promotes the production of hormones

• Promotes proper functioning of the immune system

• promotes the correct formation of the retina

• Improve the functioning of neurons and chemical transmissions

Omega 3 is probably safe for most people, including pregnant and lactating women. We recommend eating low (3 grams or less per day) dose.

Side effects that may occur:
• Belching
• Heartburn
• Nausea
• Changes in taste perception
• Back pain
• Rashes

Do not take Omega-3 before consulting your doctor if:
• Are allergic to ethyl esters or acid Omega 3 fish, including shellfish or any medications
• You are taking anticoagulants such as warfarin, aspirin or products containing, for example, treatments for hypertension, diuretics, estrogen contraceptives, etc.

• Consume more than two glasses of alcohol in one day or if you have diabetes, liver disease, thyroid or pancreas.

Theme X: L-Arginine

Arginine is a conditionally essential amino acid (is needed in the diet only under certain conditions), and may boost immune function by increasing the number of leukocytes. Arginine is involved in the synthesis of creatine, polyamines and DNA. You can lower cholesterol to improve the ability of the circulatory system and stimulate the release of growth hormone (somatropin). Arginine also reduces body fat levels and facilitates recovery of athletes because of the effects of removing ammonia (muscle resulting residue of anaerobic exercise) from the muscles and transform it into urea that is excreted in the urine. Arginine is used in the biosynthesis of creatine. It is commonly found in certain ergogenic products containing nitric oxide (NO) as power the vessel dilator effects.

How to consume L-arginine at pre-workout time : its benefits..[93]

Due to the ability of L-arginine to increase nitric oxide production and blood flow to the muscles, it is a favorite supplement among bodybuilders and is a basic ingredient in many of the pre-workout drinks. Talk to your doctor before you start taking arginine supplements. The NIH has found that arginine can interact with many different medications, including Viagra, Zantac and even over the counter medications such as aspirin and ibuprofen. Your doctor will determine if arginine supplements are safe for your condition. Do not use arginine if you are under 18, if you are pregnant or lactating. The effects of this supplement on these groups have not been widely studied.

According to the NIH guidelines, it is recommended to take 2 to 3 grams of arginine up to three times per day. Arginine supplements

---

[93] Tomado de EHow en español. obtainable in http://www.ehowenespanol.com/cuanta-larginina-debe-consumirse-del-entrenamiento-info_131344/. Accessed July 23, 2016 at 00: 23hrs.

typically come in capsule form and should be taken with a glass of water along with a meal. Since the size of arginine supplements may vary by manufacturer, follow the instructions for each product or the advice of your doctor.

JERRY BRAINUM, author of "Natural Anabolics" recommends ingesting 1.5 g of arginine an hour before exercise in order to boost the production of nitric oxide and reduce metabolic fatigue. In this way are between 0.5 to 1.5g to consume the rest of the day according to the directions above. we recommend that at least 1 g should be consumed in the morning. This way, you can consume 1 g in the morning upon waking, another quantity of 1.5 grams at half hour before exercise and, finally, 0.5 g with the last meal of the day..[94]

As a supplement, L-arginine can be taken in powder, capsule, tablet or liquid form. According BRAINUM, mixing it with grape seed extract also promote greater release of nitric oxide. The L-arginine should be taken on an empty stomach for

---

[94] This last recommendation is personal from author

best results. This eliminates the need to compete with other amino acids for absorption in the small intestine, which is the main transport system for absorption of amino acids.

Supplementation with L-arginine before exercise can produce several benefits during training sessions. L-arginine is converted to nitric oxide, an important chemical in the body plays an important role in dilating blood vessels in the regulation of blood pressure, in the release of hormones and numerous other processes. Because of this increased blood flow, more oxygen is able to reach the muscles. This allows a better supply of nutrients and reduces fatigue during training. L-arginine also helps reduce recovery time and has been supported by the most potent in promoting the release of growth hormone amino acid.

Stop taking arginine supplements if negative side effects occur. These include stomach pain, cramping and increased stool frequency. Arginine may also increase potassium levels and cause low blood pressure. Do not take arginine supplements if you are also taking ginkgo biloba supplements. Arginine may increase the risk of bleeding and it seems that the risk increases when taken along with ginkgo biloba. If you can, you try to get arginine from whole foods. Many types of nuts are good sources of arginine, especially pecans and hazelnuts. Brown rice, barley, oats and raisins are also good dietary sources of this amino acid.

Many people always ask if it is OK to drink L-arginine and creatine together. Experts believe that L-arginine contributes to improving the sanguine flow and the addition of creatine to the muscle; so many experts recommend intake both together, preferably before going to gym.

Theme XI: Casein

Casein is a type of protein that is present in milk and in some of their products, such as cheese. The main difference between casein and whey protein is its rate of absorption. Casein digests the body more slowly than whey protein. Casein is a protein rich in calcium with anti-catabolic action in the body. It is one of the basic supplements for bodybuilders, athletes and enthusiasts weightlifting. And it is important to note that one of the main protein components of animal milk, especially cattle, representing approximately 80% of total milk protein.

A hallmark of casein protein is its insolubility at low pH, such an environment would stomach acid. The slow absorption mechanism of casein is characterized by coagulation which is subjected casein when exposed to stomach acid; the resulting clot causes a slow and sustained increase in plasma amino acids. It is for this reason that casein prevents muscle catabolism. It is important to know that the anti-catabolic properties of casein is about 7-8 hours after ingestion because that time is the duration of digestion and absorption.

Casein is a protein with a very versatile use and can be used almost any time. It has the particularity that is especially useful when there are periods of time without food (such as sleep time). Furthermore, to increase the anabolic response of both proteins, it is possible to combine whey protein with casein protein. Combination for post-training in a 2 by 1 whey protein and casein protein, respectively, is ideal (eg whey protein 50gr +25gr casein protein).[95]

Each time you do a low calorie diet, one of the first issues that will become a growing concern is the loss of lean muscle mass. that happens because people do not provide enough calories to

[95] Taken from http://masamagra.com/suplementos/proteina-de-caseina-que-es-como-actua-beneficios-preguntas-frecuentes-faq/?subscribe=success#blog_subscription-2. Consulted july,23, 2016. At 21>34hrs.

fully support all energy needs throughout the day. In these cases they are forcing the body to use its own tissues for consume stored energy. In the best case, the energy required by the body will be extracted from adipose tissue of your body and in the worst case, the body will degrade muscle for obtain energy. Typically, diets of weight loss are a mixture of both.

A study in Boston tested the variations of gain lean muscle mass, as well as total fat loss, when people drank a hydrolyzate protein casein in comparison with hydrolyzed whey protein, the same time as they made a reduced calorie diet and resistance training. Although both groups showed fat loss, the group using the casein protein showed a higher average fat loss and a further increase of force on chest, shoulders and legs.

Besides this, it was also observed that the casein group left the studio with a higher percentage of total body lean mass compared to the previous measure. This indicates a higher retention rate of clean muscle mass, demonstrating that casein is especially effective in muscle maintenance.

It also should be noted that both protein groups increased their protein intake to 1.5 grams per kilogram of body weight per day.

If you are not getting enough protein while doing a diet, it will not matter what form of protein you're using, you lose muscle tissue anyway. Casein also contributes to fat loss and prevention of colon cancer.

Theme XII: BCAAs

Branched chain amino acids (BCAA) refers to a type of amino acid that has a non-linear aliphatic compound (its name comes from the characteristic branched). These include leucine, isoleucine and valine. (This is the most hydrophobic amino acids) and are ingested through proper diet. The combination of these three essential amino acids make up almost a third of the skeletal muscles in the human body and play an important role in protein synthesis. The BCAA are frequently used in the treatment of patients who have suffered burns and dietary supplements in athletes who practice bodybuilding or fitness.

One of the main functions of such amino acids is protein synthesis. BCAA oxidation metabolic whose function is to provide energy to muscles and other organs applicants it and be precursors of the synthesis of amino acids. Thus, it makes a synthesis of alanine and glutamine in states wearing catabolic, Catabolism and wearing skeletal muscle, generating a negative nitrogen balance in tissues. BCAA stops the proteolysis both in living people as in laboratory samples. This type of amino acid is taken up avidly by the muscle causing some ergogenic effects, primarily stopping the catabolic effect and promoting protein synthesis. The content of BCAA grows during the early stages of exercise and subsequently are decreasing. The reason or decay rate depends directly on the intensity of exercise.

Intake of amino acids, including BCAA, are absorbed by the small intestine via the epithelial cells through specific amino acid transporters and are transported to the liver through the bloodstream of the portal vein. BCAAs are used in the body as regulators of the synthesis and degradation (proteolysis) of proteins and are key precursor in the synthesis of alanine and glutamine. In addition, BCAA oxidation generates anaerobic energy in the muscles. BCAA oxidation is controlled, in the short term, by the products synthesized in the transamination of leucine and, in long term, by many physiological and pathological conditions such as diabetes, cancer, sepsis and infection.

It is usually ingested as a dietary supplement (often as bodybuilding supplement) in order to avoid the so-called overtraining in athletes weightlifting and bodybuilding. Its effect in reducing fatigue sport is a source of debate at present and there are scientific studies with conflicting results. It is applied as a dietary supplement in patients who have had surgery or suffering from cancer because catábolisis processes of proteins that may suffer their bodies. It has been employed as a therapy in patients suffering from dyskinesia and has been used in the meat industry as a food supplement in certain animals to obtain quality meats.

Use of BCAA as a supplement in anaerobic sports is usually done in two protocols: one drink half an hour before and another one after exercise. Some authors mention two doses, but half an hour before and 'during exercise'. Others have investigated the effect of the doses in periods prior to night rest and they claim that there is not effects on muscle growth. The BCAA are distributed in many ways, pills, powder, etc. And there are a variety of dosages ranging from one to forty grams per day. Compounds marketed typically have a ratio of 2: 1: 1 (leucine: valine: isoleucine). Some recommendations mentioned a dose of from 1.500 to 6.000 mg / day and from 800 to 3.000 mg leucine / day both isoleucine and valine. It is advised to take the branched amino acids along with protein supplements or lean meat, as well as multiple vitamins (within the group B) and minerals. 5-20 grams per day (in tablets / capsules) in divided doses during the day (some of them during exercise) or after exercise as a liquid (1 to 7 grams per liter of BCAA sports drink).

The ratio of l-leucine, l-valine and l-isoleucine with the appearance of varicocele in athletes and other unwanted effects is still being investigated.

Consuming large amounts of BCAA during exercise can decrease water absorption in the intestine which can lead to gastrointestinal problems. It is recommended to take large amounts of water during the day, from 2 to 3 liters to avoid such problems.

Theme XIII: Glycerol[96]

Glycerol is a colorless, odorless, sweet-tasting, syrupy liquid. It is 60% as sweet as sucrose and has a caloric value of 4.32 per gram. Glycerol is technically a sugar alcohol; but it could not really be considered a carbohydrate. A carbohydrate decomposes and provides some energy used in the production of lipids (fatty acids) combined together with the glycerol fatty acid triglyceride form. All carbohydrates consist of a large class of cellulose, starches and sugars. Glycerol is a natural metabolite that is rapidly absorbed and distributed throughout the body. It allows the body to temporarily retain excess fluid. This effect can help support the enlargement of muscle cells and help the effects of thermoregulation (to help prevent overheating that leads to muscle failure). Exercise can cause excessive fluid loss and glycerol can help promote hydration.

---

[96] This information has been taken from the article "How glycerol works" in the *total body building* website. Accessed on July 25, 2016.

Glycerol is part of the chemical backbone where 2 or 3 fatty acid chains are attached to create what we know as fat. Glycerin is used to make bar stay soft with the presence of proteins, trapping the water within the bar. The FDA establishes in its code of federal regulations that glycerin should be considered as a hydrate "differentiated" carbon. FDA shows this for classifying it as one of the three macro nutrients categories: fat, carbohydrates, or proteins.

A bar high in protein will have about 18 to 25 grams of glycerol in it, but will be included on the label. Too much glycerol can cause an upset stomach or diarrhea. Studies show that consuming one gram per kilo of body weight would be an exact dosage. It is recommended that does not exceed 100 grams per day.

When glycerol is administered orally, it has a moisturizing / dehydrating effect. This is based on the fact that glycerol has a capacity to hold water and can actually absorb moisture. the binding ability between water and glycerol helps keep bars very soft and also may be beneficial for endurance athletes and bodybuilders alike.

Endurance athletes can use glycerol accompanied with extra water before an event to collaborate with hydration and, therefore, improve performance. The recommended way to get the "super hydration" dose varies and each athlete must experience enough before use during the competition. For reference, we recommend you start with approximately 1 gram of glycerol per kilogram of body weight along with an additional 1.5L to 2.0L of water consumed 1 to 4 hours before the event.

We could only find five benefits of glycerol, these are::

* It is claimed that increases blood volume
* Improved temperature regulation and improved exercise performance in the heat.
* It also states that glycerol is a sweet liquid that acts like a sponge in the body.

* When consumed with water or a sports drink, glycerol causes increased fluid retention that drinking only clean water. The hyper hydration before exercise can reduce, delay or eliminate the negative effects of dehydration.

•

Bibliographic references

- Ravenstein and Hulley. 1867. *The gymnasium and its fittings* London, UK: N. Trubner and Company
- Partington, Charles F., Editor. 1838. *The British Cyclopaedia of the Arts, Sciences, History, Geography, Literature, Natural History, and Biography Volume 1 ABA to OPI* London, UK: Wm. S. Orr and Co.
- Partridge, Eric. 1984. *A Dictionary of Slang and Unconventional English.* Milton Park, Abingdon: Routledge, Taylor & Francis Group ISBN 0415065682.
- McGinn, Dave (7 November 2010). "Are protein shakes the weight-loss magic bullet?". Globe and Mail. Retrieved 1 December 2010.
- Dalby A., Food in the Ancient World A-Z, Routledge (2008) pp. 203
- A.B.A. J. 60 (1999), Hard to Swallow; Higgins, Michael
- "Are protein shakes the weight-loss magic bullet? - The Globe and Mail".

Theglobeandmail.com. Retrieved December 11, 2015.

- Spike in Harm to Liver Is Tied to Dietary Aids, The New York Times, December 21, 2013.
- "Marketplace: Some protein powders fail fitness test - Health - CBC News". Cbc.ca. Retrieved December 11, 2015.
- "Marketplace: Some protein powders fail fitness test - Health - CBC News". Cbc.ca. Retrieved December 14, 2015.
- Skip the Supplements, Paul A. Offit, chief of the division of infectious diseases at the Children's Hospital of Philadelphia, and Sarah Erush, the clinical manager in the pharmacy department of the Children's Hospital of Philadelphia. The New York Times, December 14, 2013.
- Tainted Body Building Products, FDA, December 17, 2010.
- Sports supplement designer has history of risky products, USA Today, September 27, 2013.
- Nutrition Working Group of the International Olympic Committee (2003). IOC Consensus Conference on Nutrition for Sport. Lausanne

Missing or empty |title= (help); |contribution= ignored (help)

- Dietary Reference Intakes for Energy, Carbohydrate, Fiber, Fat, Fatty Acids, Cholesterol, Protein, and Amino Acids (Macronutrients), 2005, 661.
- Journal of Sports Sciences, 2004, 22, 65–79 Protein and amino acids for athletes.
- Dietary Reference Intakes for Energy, Carbohydrate, Fiber, Fat, Fatty Acids, Cholesterol, Protein, and Amino Acids (Macronutrients), 2005, 589
- "IOC POWERADE NUTRITION WINTER - en_report_833.pdf" (PDF). Olympic.org. Retrieved December 15, 2015.

Index